Mary Regina's nursing home

WILLIAM J. BEERMAN, SR.

Supplemental information, such as audit reports and court documents from nursing home lawsuits, and post-publication developments, are available at:

https://www.wbeerman.com

Cover photos: *William Joseph Beerman;
St. Paul's Cathedral in Pittsburgh, PA;
Mary Regina Beerman; and
U.S. Steel National Works in McKeesport, PA
(National Works Photo © Courtesy of
Wonday Film Service, Wilkinsburg, PA)*

Disclaimer: The book title, **Mary Regina's nursing home**, is a generic description based on Mary Regina Beerman's real name, and it has no relationship to any similarly named nursing home or other business that may exist.

Copyright © 2017 William J. Beerman, Sr., LLC
All rights reserved.
ISBN: 978-1986310581

DEDICATION

This book is dedicated to:
- The 1.4 million people who resided in American nursing homes in 2017 -- especially those residents who, because of their exceptional longevity, family separation, or family dysfunction, found themselves alone while facing the challenges of nursing home life.
- The millions of Americans who might be headed to a nursing home, as about 10,000 American Baby Boomers turn age 65 every day from now until the year 2030.
- Those caring individuals who dedicate themselves to improving the lives of nursing home residents.
- My parents, Mary Regina Beerman and William Joseph Beerman.
- People who provided much needed encouragement as I wrote this book, including my daughter, Heidi; my son, William Jr.; editors Kathleen Smith, Sonya Weiner, and Fredric Weiner; and friend Rita Grusenmeyer.

CONTENTS

Prologue: How This Book Came To Be — i

Part 1: The Human Interest Story

Heaven has no rage like love to hatred turned,
Nor hell a fury like a woman scorned
-- English Playwright William Congreve in the "Mourning Bride," 1697

1	Early Background	1
2	Marriage and a Family	40
3	Divorce	96
4	Life After Divorce	113

Part 2: Hospitals, the Nursing Home, and a Funeral Home

Be nice to your children. After all, they are going to choose your nursing home
-- Comedian Steven Wright

5	A Broken Hip and Wrist, and Mercy Hospital	129
6	Mary Regina's Skilled Nursing Home	141
7	Western Pennsylvania Hospital, Forbes Regional Campus	171
8	A Funeral Home Hassle	177

Part 3: Government Oversight of Nursing Homes

Managers knew when inspections were coming
-- Confidential Witnesses

9	The Pennsylvania Department of Health; Inspectors Under Scrutiny	181
10	The New Mexico and Pennsylvania Attorneys General; Controversial Lawsuits; a Pornography Scandal; and a Jail Sentence	202
11	The Pennsylvania Office of the Auditor General; Now You See Them, Now You Don't	234
12	The Five-Star Rating System, and the U.S. Government Accountability Office's Audit	246
13	At National and State Levels, Consumer Complaints Rise While Citations and Enforcement Actions Decline	269
14	Nursing Home Quality Improvement Task Force Report: 1-Hour Waits for Call-Bell Responses	287
15	Advocates -- The National Consumer Voice for Quality Long-Term Care; and Problems with Nursing Home Closures	307

Epilogue: The Need for Constant Vigilance;   319
Residents *Still* in Jeopardy

Appendix A: Master's Report   333

Appendix B: Amended Bill of Particulars   342

Appendix C: Summary of Golden Living Court Decision   348

Appendix D: Private Attorneys and Nursing Homes   350

Appendix E: Remaining Questions for HHS and CMS   353

Appendix F: Examples of Supplemental Documents such as Audit Reports, a Task Force Report, and Lawsuit Briefs and Decisions Available at *https://www.wbeerman.com*   356

Prologue:
How this book came to be

I believed I was fast approaching death myself at age 67, as I reflected on the deaths of my parents. My father was only 64 when he died. But I was focused more on the death of my mother, Mary Regina, who died in Pittsburgh, PA on August 7, 2011, at the age of 86, after a stay in a nursing home.

Now it was already 2016. Mary Regina's nursing home ordeal and ultimate death had led to litigation, and I had been the prime mover for the lawsuit. Because my attorney had a low opinion of the monetary value of a wrongful death or malpractice suit about an 86-year-old woman, and lacked enthusiasm, I had to do most of the work for the lawsuit myself. I even had to change attorneys in late May 2013, just before the statute of limitations expired, because I was afraid the first attorney would fail to file suit or otherwise resolve the case before the deadline. I didn't care about the value of the case. I just wanted justice, and I did not want to forgo any course of action that might yield some justice.

Coping with my mother's illness and working on the subsequent lawsuit and this book consumed thousands of hours of what otherwise would have been peaceful and enjoyable retirement time.

I worked long, hard, and carefully on the slow-moving lawsuit, applying investigative reporting and auditing insights that I had acquired during my career. I obtained the pertinent medical records and nursing home oversight agency reports; indexed them page by page and issue by issue for the lawyer's nurse-paralegal; and spent many months reviewing and analyzing events from my mother's final days.

After the lawsuit ended, I mulled over the fact that my suit represented only one of the hundreds of thousands of human beings in America who complained that they themselves had been victims of mistreatment in nursing homes, or who felt compelled to file complaints about nursing homes on behalf of loved ones. I realized in retrospect that during the weeks I spent at my mother's bedside, I had been an inadvertent undercover shopper, or infiltrator, witnessing nursing home practices from the inside. I believed I had much more awareness about nursing home operations than most people who file complaints.

Because of what I had already seen, I decided to look further, into how government agencies oversee nursing homes. I compared my own experiences with relevant information I found in government news releases, regulations, databases, lawsuits, and audit reports. I also evaluated news releases and statistics put out by the nursing home industry, within the framework of what I had learned.

I started from the specific, my mother's case, and worked outward to the general, the state and national systems for nursing home oversight. As I wrote this book to share with others the valuable information I had gained, I also began researching the life experiences of my parents.

I wanted to humanize the statistics I found, by presenting them within the context of the lives of real people, like my family, whom the statistics represent.

As I worked on this book, I was stricken with a serious case of chemical pneumonia that hospitalized me for 5 days, at a cost of $25,000, in October 2014. The illness was

Prologue

caused by my accidental inhalation of some powdered swimming pool chlorine.

During the worst of my hospital stay, my predicament of lying in excruciating pain, at the mercy of nurses who were always busy somewhere down the hall when my hydrocodon pain killer wore off, heightened my empathy for the suffering my mother had endured.

Pneumonia was just one of a number of afflictions Mary Regina contracted in her final weeks. She went through hell. During her stay in the nursing home, I spent the days in her room, witnessing much of what happened to her during the morning and afternoon shifts, including the indignities, and listening to what she told me about the night shifts. Working from a laptop computer balanced on my knees as I sat in a chair in my mother's room, I attempted to arrange for the accommodations my mother would need after she completed her nursing home rehabilitation therapy regimen, and graduated from rehab. Unfortunately, there was to be no recovery.

***

A few months after my pneumonia ordeal, I was diagnosed with suspected heart abnormalities -- inferior and septal wall defects -- during a nuclear stress test. The pneumonia had softened up my body, wasting away 10 pounds of muscle, and unfortunately leaving the flab. I felt my health was spiraling downward and I didn't know how fast or far it would fall, or whether I could reverse the decline. As I wrote this book, I worried that the stress of thinking about the condition of my heart, and my fear of doing anything physically or mentally strenuous, would hasten my demise.

Prologue

A pensioner, I considered retirement days to be precious, and I wanted to enjoy as many as I could -- and collect as many pension checks as I could. No one could appreciate retirement life more than me.

I knew what I was giving up when I left behind my retirement lifestyle of lounging in idleness and started back to work again. My new job was to document my mother's experiences in the nursing home, and my discoveries about the government's performance as a presumed watchdog that some citizens trust to monitor nursing homes.

I had been a hard-working outstanding performer for more than 4 decades, in stressful jobs I mostly did not like. These jobs provided context for my post-employment life, making retirement feel like being free after decades in servitude to bosses who varied in competence and likeability.

I had been a newspaper reporter and an editor. Deadline pressure and other challenges kept me stressed constantly in those days.

As the only white reporter for a moderately militant black newspaper, the *New Pittsburgh Courier*, in the early Seventies, I was treated with wariness by some whites, such as businessmen, politicians, and policemen, whom I questioned about their civil rights records. I encountered mild hostility from some blacks, as I covered my assignments in the black community. Because I was white, leaders of the University of Pittsburgh's Black Student Union once shut me out of a meeting after inviting the *Courier* to cover it. This enraged my black city editor, who phoned the student leaders and cursed them out. I worked regularly with famous photographer Teenie Harris, who guided me as we covered stories in Pittsburgh

Prologue

neighborhoods such as the Hill District and Homewood-Brushton, where few white people dared to go.

As managing editor of the financially constrained *Monongahela Daily Herald* in southwestern Pennsylvania coal country during 1977 and 1978, I would walk a few blocks up Main Street from my apartment and open the paper's front door at 5 a.m. each weekday. I would walk back home 10 or 12 hours later after a hectic day at work, as 30-ton coal trucks lumbered noisily past me along Main Street. Although I was chronically fatigued, I had trouble sleeping as I worried about stories the paper would publish or had already published. I wondered, how angry would the people written about be?

I encountered anger up close when emotional coal miners pushed me and the paper's photographer through a crowd and ejected us out the door from a United Mine Workers strike meeting.

There also were routine daily worries and hassles for me at the *Daily Herald*. Were there any mistakes in the police news? Would I be sued for libel? I would get phone calls at my desk with nasty salutations such as, "What the hell is wrong with you people down there?" I even worried about whether I had checked to make sure the union typographers had put the correct date in the logo on the day's front page, which once, they didn't. That day the publisher, Jack Schiffer, left a copy of the paper on my desk, with a circle around the erroneous date and the initials, JS, in red.

Resources were insufficient to do the job right and I had to fill much of the paper with cheap copy from the United Press International wire service machine that typed away prolifically behind my desk. I was fighting a losing battle as I tried to put out a respectable newspaper. I had heard that Schiffer fired the former editor without notice, on a Friday, after secretly arranging in advance for me to take over the editor's desk the following Monday morning. I knew I could be fired the same way.

While suffering at the *Daily Herald*, I was very happy to receive an offer of a public affairs job on the staff of a two-star general at the Defense Logistics Agency. I took the job even though it meant relocating my family 300 miles to Philadelphia. I reasoned that I needed to rest for a while in a secure, slow-paced "government job" before returning to newspaper work some day.

But the general's executive officer, an Army Ranger lieutenant colonel, did not like my boss, the public affairs officer, and the "XO" made things difficult for the Public Affairs Office. Then, after a black general assumed command and the public affairs officer, who was white, clashed with the black EEO (equal employment opportunity) officer and decided to quit, I changed jobs too.

Continuing my career journey from one stressful job to another, I took what I naively expected would be an easy job working for a Navy captain as an editor of audit reports for the U.S. Naval Audit Service (NAVAUD), the Department of the Navy's (DON's) 500-auditor internal audit organization. While at NAVAUD, I oversaw a staff of five technical editors, completed the required 24 credits of accounting and related courses in night school, and passed the rigorous 2-day exam to become a certified internal auditor.

My job as the auditor general's gatekeeper for his audit reports put me into conflict with audit managers. The managers wanted their audit reports, which usually were

Prologue

already late, to clear editing and be released fast. But the auditor general's top priority was that the reports comply with government auditing standards for reporting, and he relied on me and my staff to make sure they did. I was in the middle of a deliberately designed conflict situation and I spent many years arguing with audit managers and their teams over problems with hundreds of different audit findings, sometimes during grueling trips to audit sites scattered across the U.S. or in Europe.

While at NAVAUD, I took a second job, moonlighting as a stringer (correspondent) for the *Philadelphia Inquirer's* South Jersey edition. I wrote hundreds of byline stories, many of them nerve-wracking night-time stories filed right at deadline, for the morning paper. I hoped, in vain, that someday I would get back into the newspaper business full-time by landing a Newspaper Guild job with the prestigious Pulitzer Prize-winning *Inquirer*, whose multiple levels of editors relentlessly enforced high standards on virtually every story.

Contrary to my early expectations, none of my Department of Defense (DOD) "government jobs," including the one in DON, turned out to be easy, primarily because I tried to do them well.

My most demanding job by far was for an agency that literally may not be named. That job came at the end of my career. Because of a nondisclosure agreement I had signed, I was required to submit the paragraphs describing this job to a DOD agency for pre-publication review. I had to wait 28 weeks for the ultimate reply to my request for a "pre-pub." The following censored text was approved for publication with mandatory redactions -- including deletion of the name of the agency -- and the reviewer's suggested alternative wording (shown in brackets).

Prologue

The changes were imposed not because the original text compromised classified information, but because it contained information that was "determined" to be "inappropriate for public release," according to the reviewer. The agency also required that the following disclaimer be published: "All assertions of fact and opinion are those of the author and do not reflect the policy or position of the Department of Defense or its components or the U.S. Government."

The job spanned 8 years of evening and night shifts [ONE LINE REMOVED] in the basement of the Pentagon, where I worked as one of the editors for the [DEPARTMENT OF DEFENSE].

[FIVE LINES REMOVED]

Mistakes [WORDS REMOVED] were not acceptable, and the [PRODUCT I EDITED] had to be out each morning at 5:30 [ONE LINE REMOVED]. The [PRODUCT] had to be approved by "the J2," a general or admiral who was the top military intelligence officer for the Joint Chiefs of Staff [WORDS REMOVED]. The J2 directorate is the [WORDS REMOVED] focal point for crisis intelligence support to military operations, among other roles. The last J2 that I worked under was sometimes blustery, and most of the half-dozen or so intelligence analysts who briefed him in a formal setting around a conference table at "o five hundred" each morning probably were a little afraid of him. Everyone stood up when the J2 entered the room.

The J2 did not care about the deadline if he decided to make last-minute changes in the day's [PRODUCT], but I still had to get the changes made by 5:30. [THREE LINES REMOVED] Sometimes the atmosphere was so tense that I could not afford to waste 15 or 30 seconds so I ignored the

Prologue

ringing phone as my fingers flew across my keyboard or I carefully reviewed a checklist, and individual sentences, [WORDS REMOVED], with my full attention meticulously focused in on each word, one at a time, in sequence.

Besides feeling the deadline pressure, I knew that [FOUR LINES REMOVED]. When [THE SENIOR EDITOR] was on extended sick leave or vacation, I was responsible for guiding the staff, coordinating with article authors, compiling and reviewing the [PRODUCT], getting it to the J2, and having it properly disseminated.

It seemed to me that catching every single one of the potential errors or security violations that might slip by the [WORD REMOVED] editorial and graphics staffers, despite the internal control system in place, was impossible over the long run. I felt as though a catastrophe always was hovering over my head, threatening to fall like the Sword of Damocles. Each evening when I reported to work, I worried that I would be told that a security violation had occurred the night before and that I was to be questioned during a mandatory investigation. Fortunately, by exercising utmost caution and working in a constant state of hypertension, I succeeded in preventing any security violation on my watch.

The Intelligence Community during my years with [DOD] took information security much more seriously than the State Department apparently did under Secretary Hillary Clinton. [EIGHT LINES REMOVED]

In 2004, I volunteered for a 6-month deployment to Baghdad to help write reports. While *en* route there in October, I was stopped short in Qatar, where I served as the DOD civilian employee chief of a team of contractors writing information reports from captured Iraqi documents.

Prologue

During my deployment, which I completed in April 2005, I lived in a converted Kormax shipping container shared with one other occupant and worked in a prefab office surrounded by chain link fencing in an air conditioned warehouse on an Army camp in the desert. I flew to Baghdad twice to coordinate my team's efforts for the information needs in Iraq.

While deployed, I encountered multiple workplace conflicts, and at one point I came to realize that no matter what unpleasantness I might encounter during the rest of my career, I would always be able to console myself with the thought, "At least I am not in Qatar."

I told my doctor about my stress on the job, and the doctor prescribed Atenolol, a beta blocker blood pressure medication. Nearly burned out, I retired from the Pentagon job in the J2 Directorate at my first opportunity, with 30 years' service in DOD, on the very day of my 60th birthday, October 1, 2008.

I absolutely <u>loved</u> that I did not have to go to work anymore. I simply could not believe how lucky I was. The pension I earned during more than 4 decades in the world of work in private industry and government seemed almost worth the workplace trials and tribulations, in hindsight. I could have enhanced my pension by working longer, but I was certain that by retiring and leaving the stress behind, I had extended my life expectancy. I had no regrets about retiring.

I wanted time to pass slowly so I could savor my freedom.

In retirement, in sunny New Mexico, I spent parts of those lazy days leisurely skimming out rose petals that

Prologue

breezes blew into my backyard pool. I smugly asked myself, "Does life get any better than this?"

I measured time not by looking ahead to weekends as a typical worker might, but by keeping track of garbage days. Tuesday was the day the garbage truck came down my street in my retirement town of Las Cruces, NM, and I had to wheel my garbage container to the curb. This was one of few demands on me in my life as a pensioner. I could pretty much do whatever I wanted, whenever I wanted, as long as it wasn't too expensive.

But it seemed that <u>every</u> day was Tuesday, Garbage Day, the weeks went by so fast. I wondered, "What happened to Wednesday through Monday?" Time was blowing by like those cliché calendar pages that the wind whisked away in an old Turner Classic movie to show the passage of months or even years in 5 seconds of movie time.

The precious, blissful days of retirement after a hard life at work were vaporizing. I felt they would be gone in a flash. When I was 65, I told my son, William John, Jr., "You know, I've already lived longer than your grandfather (William Joseph). I am living on borrowed time."

My parents, who had little else in common after the end of their disastrous marriage, both, astonishingly, suffered heart attacks within 2 days of each other in January, 1990, when they were both 64 years old. I was visiting my mother in Pittsburgh's Mercy Hospital, where she had been taken after collapsing in a restaurant because of a heart attack, when I received a phone call at the nurses' station. In that stunning call, my Aunt Jean told me that my father had died of a sudden, massive heart attack at Conch Key, in the Florida Keys. "You're kidding," was my clumsy reply. Mary Regina survived her heart attack, had a pacemaker implanted, and lived on for 2 more decades.

My mother and I never had a good relationship. Instead, Mary Regina shared her life with my 9-year-younger sister, Jeanne. When Mary Regina left my father several times in the Sixties to go home to her parents, she took young Jeanne with her. I remember my mother once inviting me to come along as she walked out the door with my sister and the family dog. But despite the invitation, we both knew I would not go with her.

After Jeanne grew up and married, Mary Regina joined my sister's family -- her daughter, son-in-law, and two grandchildren -- who welcomed her warmly for extended visits to their homes, first, in Michigan, and then in Oregon. They treated her with respect, took her on their many vacations, and loved her. When Mary Regina was home in Pittsburgh, my sister and her family stayed in close touch through regular phone calls, and Jeanne looked after Mary Regina.

When Jeanne died at age 52 in 2009 of metastacized breast cancer, Mary Regina's world began melting down, and my idle retirement life was over for a while. I found myself assuming responsibility as my mother's sole surviving "issue" – the term the Pennsylvania Orphans Court uses to designate a son or daughter. Mary Regina not only found herself bereft of her daughter, but her ability to live independently, and even her desire to live at all, were fading rapidly.

Mary Regina was suddenly in the awkward position of being somewhat dependent upon a son with whom she had a strained relationship and who had moved 1,775 miles away.

Prologue

Mary Regina's decline and death forced a multiyear hiatus in my carefree retirement and renewed the stress on me. I had to try to arrange accommodations for my less than cooperative mother in my own home or an assisted living facility. I had to cope on the fly with her sudden hospitalization for a broken hip and wrist, her dreadful stay in a skilled nursing rehabilitation facility, her emergency transfer to another hospital, and her ultimate death. I subsequently felt compelled to expose, and seek justice for, the mistreatment she suffered, and to share my experiences with others who might find my accounts usefully informative.

At the end of it all, in my waning years, I don't fear death, but I fear a horrible protracted pre-death ordeal such as my mother suffered. I don't want to get trapped in a substandard nursing home. When the New Mexico Supreme Court ruled on July 1, 2016 that doctor-assisted death is not a fundamental liberty in my state, I was disappointed and began hoping the New Mexico state legislature would enact a law that supplants the court decision.

TO SKIP THE HUMAN-INTEREST BACKGROUND STORY
ABOUT MARY REGINA AND ME, GO TO PART TWO

PART ONE: The Human Interest Story

*Heaven has no rage like love to hatred turned,
Nor hell a fury like a woman scorned*
—English playwright William Congreve in
"The Mourning Bride"

Chapter 1: Early Background

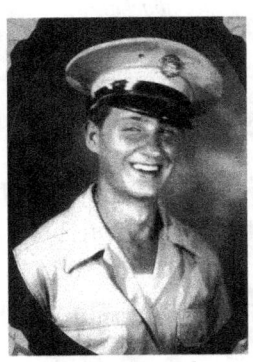

William Joseph Beerman during World War II

William Joseph Beerman, my father, and Mary Regina Beerman, nee Fisher, my mother, were born in 1925, grew up during the Great Depression, and matured into adulthood during World War II.

They came from different backgrounds. My mother had the University of Pittsburgh's Cathedral of

1

Chapter 1: Early Background

Learning in her back yard, figuratively speaking, and my father probably had an outhouse in his.

My father, who was poor during the Depression, dropped out of high school in 1942 during the tenth grade to go to work, but soon became a teenage soldier. For the first half of 1944 he was billeted with a family in Swansea, Wales, United Kingdom. After being shipped across the English Channel to Normandy shortly after D-Day, he spent the second half of 1944 and part of 1945 in France as the allied armies were driving the Germans back to Germany.

In some respects, my father would become an exemplary member of the "Greatest Generation." He was not a war hero. But aspects of his life might serve well as a model for members of succeeding generations, such as his children, who were Baby Boomers, and his grandchildren and great-grandchildren, who are part of Generations X, Y, and Z.

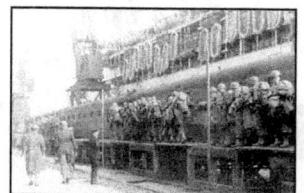

American troops disembarking at the Swansea dock

Mary Regina had a childhood to be envied by many of her contemporaries during the Depression. The comfortable days of her youth from the late 1920s through the mid-1940s culminated after the war in a storybook romance with a returning soldier who moved in next-door, and a marriage that seemingly was made in heaven. But her sweet love relationship would sour quickly and her marriage to my father would evolve into a marriage from hell that generated unhappiness for decades for Mary Regina and her family.

Chapter 1: Early Background

Later, in a second cruel blow from life, my mother's old age in the Third Millennium would end in a death that could only be described as a merciful answer to her prayers -- and vocal pleading -- that she be released from emotional and physical agony and be allowed to die.

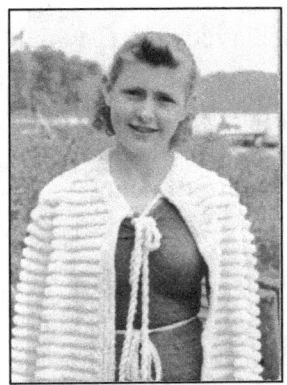

Mary Regina, age 16, on vacation at lake-side in 1941

Mary Regina grew up in Oakland, the urban cultural center of Pittsburgh. At the heart of Oakland was the University of Pittsburgh's Cathedral of Learning, a gothic revival, 42-story tower that is the tallest education building in the Western Hemisphere. The edifice was dedicated in 1937, when Mary Regina was 12, and Mary Regina could see it from outside her home about a dozen blocks away. She eventually would send her daughter to "Pitt," where Jeanne would get her master's degree in education and meet Mary Regina's future son-in-law, a graduate engineering student.

Mary Regina and her family could walk from their home to the Oakland cultural campus built by Scotsman Andrew Carnegie, the founder of U.S. Steel Corporation.

The Carnegie complex was a window to the world for Pittsburghers -- a superb repository and exhibition venue

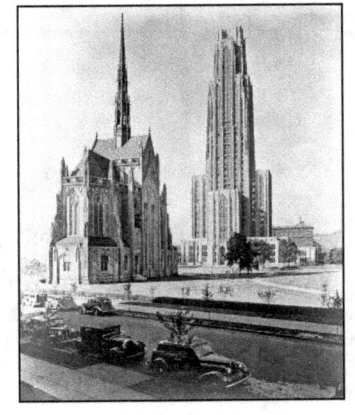

University of Pittsburgh 42-story tower with Pitt's Heinz Chapel in the foreground, in the 1930s.
Photo: Carnegie Library of Pittsburgh, Pa. Dept.

Chapter 1: Early Background

for knowledge and the arts. It included Carnegie Museum of Natural History, Carnegie Museum of Art, Carnegie Library and Institute of Pittsburgh, and Carnegie Music Hall. The museum of natural history had, for example, the world's finest collection of dinosaur fossils. The earliest creature in the collection was the spectacular *Diplodocus* Carnegie, a 90-foot-long skeleton, displayed erect, which made its Pittsburgh debut in 1907. Size was no deterrent for Carnegie's curators. They even exhibited within their halls examples of ancient Greek and Roman architecture that Andrew Carnegie shipped in from the Mediterranean.

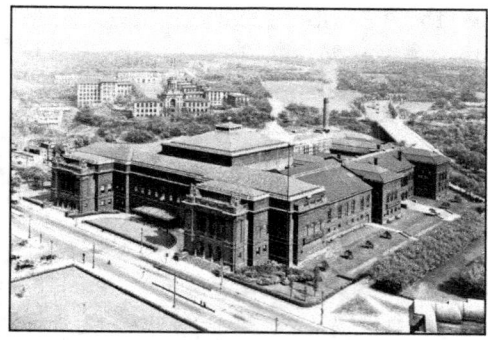

Carnegie Library and Institute, with Carnegie Institute of Technology (now Carnegie Mellon University) in the upper left background, in 1937.
Photo: Carnegie Library of Pittsburgh, Pa. Dept.

Oakland was the setting for the ballet academy later portrayed as the classy conservatoire that intimidated aspiring dance student Jennifer Beals in the 1983 movie *Flash Dance*. Forbes Field, the former home of the Pittsburgh Pirates baseball team, was in Oakland. And the Phipps Conservatory and Botanical Gardens were nearby in Schenley Park. In the Oakland-Shadyside-Squirrel Hill district, particularly along Fifth Avenue, stood mansions where some of Pittsburgh's industrialists once lived.

Mary Regina lived at 3301 Ward Street, in a freestanding single-family corner house in a modest Oakland neighborhood near Schenley Park.

Chapter 1: Early Background

She attended St. Paul's Cathedral Catholic high school for girls on North Craig Street, where she must have mingled with young ladies from some of Pittsburgh's higher echelon families. She was an average student in the business track with progressively better grades each year, a grade-point average of 83 as a senior, and ordinary intelligence quotient (IQ) scores of 102, 97, and 107 in 1940, 1941, and 1943, respectively. She missed only 1 day of school in 4 years, and she was ranked 40th in a class of 72 when she graduated on June 6, 1943. Her economic status was checked off as "average" on her permanent record.

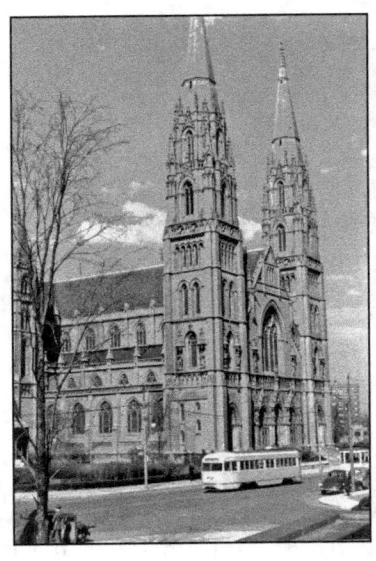

St Paul's Cathedral, 1940, while Mary Regina was a student at Cathedral High
Photo: Carnegie Library of Pittsburgh, Pa. Dept.

During her high school years Mary Regina looked as pretty and delicate as a flower. But later, in a 13-year divorce war, she would emerge as a tough, ruthless menace for her beleaguered husband and she certainly was the main character in his nightmares.

Despite her combat experience as a divorce warrior and her battle-hardened persona, she would be as helpless as a lamb in the world of a nursing home during the last days of her life.

John Aloysius Fisher, Mary Regina's father, as the Cathedral High School records assessed, was not affluent -- just "average," financially. But during the Depression Era

Chapter 1: Early Background

of the 1930s, he was fortunate enough to have a steady job for the "P&LE" -- the Pennsylvania and Lake Erie Railroad -- while some Pittsburghers stood in soup lines or lived in shantytowns like Hooverville, on Liberty Avenue, less than 2 miles north of the Cathedral of Learning.

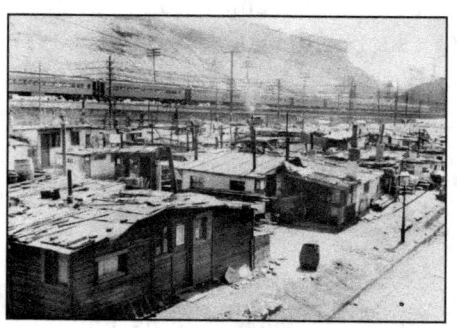

Pittsburgh's Depression-Era shantytown, Hooverville, on Liberty Avenue
Photo: Carnegie Library of Pittsburgh, Pa. Dept.

John Fisher was born on January 23, 1897 in Carnegie, PA, near Pittsburgh, and according to the 1920 Census, John's father, Samuel P. Fisher, was a general foreman for the P&LE. As years went by, John progressed through jobs as crossing flagman and engineer's helper, to track gang foreman. He worked out of the P&LE terminal yard at Carson and Smithfield Streets, in Pittsburgh's South Side, which now is a tourist attraction called Station Square.

I have knowledge about my grandparents John and Agnes Fisher, in the form of childhood memories I accumulated during the Fifties and early Sixties, when I spent time each week at the home to which they moved in Dormont Borough, on the City of Pittsburgh's southern border. Because of my memories, I can infer what Mary Regina's early life with John and Agnes had been like.

John was a man of exceptional refinement for a working man although at times he expressed opinions that some today might consider to be very politically incorrect.

Chapter 1: Early Background

John took me on tours of the Carnegie complex when I was a child; he frequented libraries in Oakland and elsewhere; and he was a history aficionado. He was fond of classical music such as Tchaikovsky's War of 1812 Overture, especially the rendition performed with sound effects, including real cannon fire, by the Boston Pops Orchestra. He had it on an LP record album that he played on his Hi-Fi for my father and me. John could relate the movements of the overture to events in the war, such as the reputed playing of *La Marseillaise*, the French National Anthem, in a futile effort to rally Napoleon's troops, and the joyous pealing of church bells to proclaim the defeat of the invaders of Mother Russia.

My grandfather had discretionary income as I was growing up, some of which he used for vacations. He took my father and me on educational trips to Washington, DC, to George Washington's home at Mount Vernon, VA, and to the Gettysburg Civil War battlefield in south-central Pennsylvania. He brought me with him for a week-long fishing vacation at an island camp in Parry Sound, Ontario, Canada. There, we were caught, in a 12-foot boat, completely out of sight of land, by an unforgettably frightening storm that blew up on the sound. I don't understand how, but John managed to find his way back to the dock through 4-foot crests and troughs. During less exciting days of this vacation, we fished from the dock for bait fish. We fried Northern Pike on a black cast iron woodstove in our cabin and ate it for breakfast, lunch, and dinner.

John earned sufficient money that he could invest in some gold coins, which he kept wrapped in Kleenex in his desk.

Chapter 1: Early Background

He served for the family at Sunday dinners fare such as lobster Newburg, lamb with mint jelly, and sauerbraten. As an after-dinner drink, he liked Heering Cherry Liqueur.

The food was prepared by John's tiny Scotch-Irish wife, my grandmother, Agnes, *nee* Conoly (who was measured at 4-foot-10 at age 83). She was an intelligent woman, with a kind nature, who reminded me of a smaller and quieter version of Archie Bunker's wife Edith, the character in the Seventies TV show *All in the Family*.

Agnes had all the skills and the proper personality necessary to qualify as one of the world's best grandmothers.

My grandmother did her cooking and baking from scratch, using her crank-driven metal flour sifter and manual egg beater, and other now rarely seen kitchen utensils. For her apple pies, she would core and peel and slice the apples, roll out the dough with her wooden or metal rolling pins, and add in the apples, lemon juice, cinnamon, and Land o' Lakes butter pats.

With the leftover raw pie dough that she trimmed from the rims of her Pyrex glass pie plates, she would make 2-inch cinnamon-and-sugar spiral rolls, which she would bake with the pies and offer to me as treats. Cakes in the Fisher home also were made from the basic ingredients, and I knew that John disapproved of "box cake."

I would hang out in the kitchen with my grandmother, drinking hot chocolate, Coca Cola, Pepsi, or Hires Root Beer, and eating Cheez-Its, M&M'S, HERSHEY'S Miniatures, or a Klondike ice cream bar. Agnes made hot chocolate with real HERSHEY'S cocoa and sugar, not with instant chocolate milk mix.

Chapter 1: Early Background

My grandmother's house was immaculate and washing down all the walls with buckets of Spic AND Span cleaner and big natural sponges was a spring cleaning ritual. She put the males of the family to work for this task. There were no cobwebs anywhere in the house -- not even in the basement.

Agnes ironed everything. She had down in the basement a mangle ironing machine, which had a padded roller that was heated and turned by electricity. She used it to press the bedsheets and tablecloths. The sheets would smell fresh, and feel crisp and cool when I would crawl into bed in a spare bedroom during sleepovers. Agnes had other homemaking equipment in the basement such as a sewing machine with a foot treadle made of ornate cast iron lattice, a wringer washer, and wooden stretcher frames with rows of needles spaced every half-inch to hold curtains and drapes taut after washing so they dried without shrinking. Clothes lines were strung among the joists in the basement, and the hung laundry dripped a few drops of water onto a smooth concrete floor that was coated with shiny dark-red paint, probably the now-outlawed poisonous type of paint known then as "red lead."

Agnes shopped for quality merchandise, including gifts for me, downtown at the Kaufman's, Gimbels, and Joseph Horne's department stores. She brought home on the streetcar shopping bags containing articles of new clothing folded into glossy red or white gift boxes lined with tissue paper.

Grandma Agnes doted on me, her first grandchild.

However, the disharmony between my mother and me already was emerging when I was only 3 or 4 years old. Grandma would admonish my mother when Mary Regina

Chapter 1: Early Background

treated me harshly. "Oh Jeanie!" Agnes would scold her daughter, if Mary Regina did or said something nasty to me, such as warning me about interrupting the adults' conversation ("Children are to be seen, and not heard," Mary Regina would say), or snatching away my annoying Fisher-Price "Corn Popper" toy. The contraption, which is still sold today, had a dozen wooden balls that popped loudly against a plastic dome in rapid fire as a kid pulled or pushed it by its wooden handle on its wheels.

Thinking about my relationships with my grandmother and mother, I was reminded of humorist Sam Levenson's quote: "The reason grandparents and grandchildren get along so well is that they have a common enemy."

On many Sundays during the late Fifties and early Sixties as I grew older, Agnes would give me a quarter or 35 cents for the movies, where I would see horror films such as *The Tingler* with Vincent Price and *The Blob* with Steve McQueen; westerns; Doris Day films; *The Horse Soldiers,* a Civil War story with John Wayne; and Audrey Hepburn in *The Nun's Story*. Agnes sent me to the movies because she knew I would not be happy if I had to stay cooped up with the adults all day.

I noticed that Agnes sometimes would just sit and stare at me, admiringly and lovingly. Later, I would think of Agnes when I heard the Paul Simon song, *Loves Me Like a Rock*:

> *My mama loves me.*
> *She loves me.*
> *She gets down on her knees and hugs me.*
> *She loves me like a rock.*

In my mind I would substitute the word "grandma" for "mama." That made the lyrics true.

Chapter 1: Early Background

***

Although Grandfather John's job as a track gang foreman primarily was an outdoor job, he prepared first-line supervisor's reports at home. John would sit in his suspenders and plaid shirt, with the sleeves rolled up, exposing his wool long underwear top, and make out his reports in exquisite cursive handwriting on yellow legal-pad paper and pale green graph paper. He would work at the dining room table or at his polished secretary in an upstairs room set up as an office. In his desk's pigeonholes and drawers of various sizes were fountain pens, ink bottles, a stapler, scissors, and other office articles that I found alluring.

Exploring the desk when no one was around, engrossed in my own world of a child, I would work my mischievous little fingers to twist off the cap of an ink bottle, or take apart the fountain pens, which had rubber bladders inside, and the mechanical pencils, which had screw-driven devices to adjust the lead. I would become so absorbed that my keen young olfactory senses discerned the subtle scents emanating from the desk's green felt blotter, the box of graphite refills for the mechanical pencils, the ink in the bottle, and the rubbery gum block erasers. If anyone would have entered the room and begun watching me, I would have been oblivious to their presence.

Outside the office on the hallway wall hung a large copy of the classic painting *Scottish Boy with Wolfhounds* by James Jnr Hardy. The scene with a kid and dogs, of course, attracted my notice.

John Fisher's house was brick over terracotta tile block. The building was solid and quiet. It was cool in the summer in those days before residential air conditioning.

Chapter 1: Early Background

When there was snow outside, the coal furnace in the cellar and a hot-water radiator in each room kept the house warm.

I subconsciously felt that my grandparents' world was far more pleasant, comfortable, interesting, and secure than my own in Port Vue, Pennsylvania, 13 miles down the Monongahela River in the Steel Valley.

John Fisher was a success and he had established an excellent home.

***

John's neck was red. The back of it was quilted into hairy one-inch squares separated by deep crevices. This tanned alligator hide was a result of years out on the railroad tracks around Pittsburgh in places like Homestead, Braddock, Rankin, and West Newton in the frigid wind of winter and the strong sun of summer.

John spent the majority of his waking hours each workday with a track gang that included Negro men, who John said possessed impressive skill for driving 6-inch spikes with sledgehammers, and strength for hefting, as a team, 500-pound steel rails and 200-pound creosoted wooden railroad ties, and for shoveling gravel roadbed ballast. This work was becoming mechanized as technology advanced during the 1950s. Maintaining railroads required more than spikes, rails, and ties. The work utilized a veritable storehouse of specialized track hardware, tools, and mobile equipment. It demanded knowledge of blueprints, track creep, drainage, train schedules, and safety protocols.

John expressed opinions that would explode the heads of today's thought and speech police. He served from March 1918 to June 1919 as a Doughboy private first class

Chapter 1: Early Background

in the 32nd Engineers in France, as part of the American Army that fought the Germans in World War I. But some of his prejudices faintly reflected those associated with stereotypical Germans of the Thirties and Forties.

John, an ethnic German himself, would not have supported harming Jews, and he certainly didn't hate them, but he harbored an unfavorable opinion about the ethnic group. He had a copy of Adolf Hitler's book, *Mein Kampf*, and he could quote it. He had read the *Merchant of Venice*, Shakespeare's play in which a Jewish moneylender demands a pound of flesh from a debtor. He voiced slurs about Jews, and although John was fond of some black members of his track crew, he slurred blacks too. Today, many people might not recognize some of John's racially and ethnically derogatory words. I learned a number of them at a young age from my grandfather.

Later, as a young liberal Democrat who admired assassinated President John F. Kennedy, I graduated from Penn State School of Journalism in 1970 and got a job as the only white employee at Pittsburgh's somewhat prestigious, century-old, black newspaper, *The New Pittsburgh Courier*. After hearing about my new job, John bluntly asked me, "Why are you working for that n----- newspaper?"

To be fair, I cannot recall John ever using actual "swear words," such as goddamn or shit, and in his defense, racial and ethnic prejudices were quite common for the times. My Dad, for example, would tell me not to play "n----- music" on the car radio. He observed that Port Vue, the town where I grew up, was populated largely by "hunkies" – meaning eastern Europeans such as Czechs, Serbs, Slovaks, Poles, and Hungarians, many of whom worked in the steel mills, and who were also sometimes

Chapter 1: Early Background

called "mill hunks." Italians, too, had their special names. Mary Regina would casually ask Dad to bring home a loaf of "Dago bread" to go with a Chef Boyardee spaghetti dinner.

The display case at the penny candy store I visited as a kid had black licorice jelly candies called "n----- toes" and "n----- babies" during the late Fifties and early Sixties.

I knew from working at the *Courier* that some blacks called some other blacks n-----s, or Oreos, after the cookies (black on the outside, white on the inside), and that some blacks called some whites "honkeys." There even was some prejudice implicit in the fact that my black militant city editor boss Diane Perry told me I was "a good white," implying that many whites, if not most, were not good.

But John's prejudices seemed relatively strong, and he would lecture his son-in-law in living room monologues about race and ethnicity as his young grandson listened in. John's were the dominant voice and personality in his home.

When Grandma Agnes died on August 1, 1997 at the age of 92, I was quite surprised to hear my mother say that Agnes did not want to be buried in the same plot at Queen of Heaven Cemetery as John, who had preceded her in death in 1984 at the age of 87. I was amused, to my shame, that they buried her there anyway. I realized then that if you become incapacitated and dependent upon others, as a resident of a nursing home, for example, or, of course, if you die, it might not be <u>thy</u> will that be done, but the will of someone else.

Chapter 1: Early Background

Possibly Agnes's direction about her last resting place was influenced more by her old age than by John's true deportment as a husband and a person.

I had information from Mary Regina about "family strife" and Agnes's relationship with Mary Regina when Agnes was in her eighties. Agnes reportedly had an "inability to get along peacefully with her children," had a distant relationship with John, and blamed John for many of her problems. It occurred to me later that my mother seemed to share some of these traits with my grandmother, but they emerged at a younger age in Mary Regina's case.

So, to give John the benefit of the doubt about his domestic manners would not necessarily be wrong.

John did some nice things. He gave to me when I was 18 his 1955 Plymouth after he got to be too old to drive it, and he took in my sister Jeanne when our parents split up. John helped make sure Jeanne got through high school and college. He gave her away at her wedding, because her father was not welcome at his girl's wedding and he had to have the ceremony surreptitiously videotaped by a well-meaning wedding crasher who, thank goodness, did not get caught. I thought John might have paid for the wedding, which was a nice one.

Ironically, John displayed admirable behavior by taking care of my sister, but he collaborated -- possibly unwittingly -- with my vindictive mother as she cruelly alienated my sister from our father, who loved her dearly. Jeanne was deprived of having a father in her life, and of knowing her father's side of the family. Today's popular word, "enabler," might be accurately descriptive of John's role in supporting my mother's inappropriate behavior.

***

Chapter 1: Early Background

Mary Regina and her siblings were not exceptionally small like Agnes. I wondered whether John periodically gave them glasses of water with drops of iodine in them to drink, as he did with me. John believed this would stimulate my thyroid gland and make me grow taller.

Mary Regina had two brothers, who were proper people, and their behavior possibly made Mary Regina think my conduct was unsatisfactory compared to that of her brothers. Similarly, Grandfather John had been an altar boy, and Mary Regina was very disappointed when the nuns who ran my elementary school declined to pick me to be an altar boy, even though Mary Regina asked them to. She wanted me to wear the same altar boy cassock her father had worn as a child. But Mary Regina's son, unlike her father, simply was not altar boy material, in the estimation of the nuns. Looking back as an old man, I wondered why, although I didn't care much.

One of Mary Regina's brothers, called Jack or Junior, was born about 1927. He went off to World War II as a seaman in the South Pacific, and survived. According to Mary Regina, he wanted so badly to get into the service that he hung by his hands from doorframes, stretching himself to ensure he could meet the Navy's height requirement. In his uniform he looked trim and fit in wartime photographs. As he aged, Jack, an employee of the P&LE Railroad, developed a masculine image. He smoked stogies, and sometimes wore a big ring of keys that hung from the belt loop of his Big Mac-style khaki pants.

The younger brother, Bobby, born about 1931, still lived with my grandparents when I was a child, allowing for a slight overlap of our generations and some interaction between Bobby and me.

Chapter 1: Early Background

Bobby epitomized an ideal young man in my view. Bobby didn't have a brother named Beaver, but he had Wally Cleaver's perfect personality, as portrayed in the TV series, *Leave it to Beaver*, which aired from 1957 to 1963. The show portrayed a model American family, in which mature and well-balanced high school student Wally helped guide his naïve little brother, grade schooler Beaver, out of jams. Beaver's predicaments often were caused by Wally's nasty friend Eddie Haskell. Wikipedia today says that the character Eddie Haskell "has become a cultural reference, recognized as an archetype for insincere sycophants." The Wikipedia article calls Eddie two-faced, sneaky, shallow, conniving, and weaselly. I was influenced by one or two Eddie Haskell types in my own life but to my misfortune I did not have an older brother like Wally to guide me.

If Eddie Haskell was a "cultural reference" for a dislikeable kid, Wally Cleaver was a cultural reference for a nice young man, like my Uncle Bobby.

Bobby attended Dormont High School, which I thought looked just like Wally Cleaver's idyllic high school. Later I would choose to live in Haddon Heights, NJ, and send my kids to Haddon Heights High, partly because the town and school were reminiscent of Dormont and Dormont High. I believed Haddon Heights was the ideal place to raise kids.

As a young man, Bobby drove a big, new, Simonized green and white 1958 Plymouth with fins. Mary Regina called it "the boat."

As Bobby played 45-rpm records of Fifties music, he would tell me, "Down, not up," advising that a smoothed-down Princeton hair style was preferable to the wavy slicked-back "greaser" style, later worn on TV by "the

Chapter 1: Early Background

Fonz" in *Happy Days*. He also told me that black socks and cordovan penny loafers were preferable to white socks with black shoes and pants. Uncle Bobby was too nice to use the word greaser. That is my word.

Bobby was drafted into the Army during the Korean War. The night he left, his mother Agnes lay face down on the sofa bawling inconsolably, "Why my Bobby? Why my Bobby?" He was his mother's favorite, Mary Regina said, and Mary Regina criticized Bobby for moving later in life 300 miles away to Eastern Pennsylvania, outside Philadelphia, with his pretty wife, Shirley, and later to Florida, leaving his mother behind. Notably, I would move 1,775 miles away from my mother, Mary Regina, when I grew up.

Fortunately for my grandmother, she would not have to worry too much about Bobby during the Korean War, because he served his Army time as a medic in Alabama, rather than in Korea where he could have ended up in a M*A*S*H unit (mobile Army surgical hospital) like the one in the TV series and movie. I think I remember my mother saying Uncle Bobby was a conscientious objector, but I am not sure. Bobby gave me an Army medic's hand brush with the caduceus embossed on it, the kind of brush that operating room teams used to scrub up. I felt a strange admiration for the unusual implement and was proud of my uncle. Bobby was selected as my first communion sponsor.

After the Army, Bobby got a job with a railroad, the Seaboard, which ran along the Atlantic Coast, but, unlike his father, he had an office job. Mary Regina told me that Bobby was a "male secretary." Later, judging by the fact that Bobby reportedly had converted a barn into a very nice house, I figured Bobby probably had a higher paying job than secretary. As Bobby reached middle age, he looked

Chapter 1: Early Background

like actor Jack Lemmon when Lemmon played an executive in the 1970 movie, *The Out-of-Towners*.

From what I gathered from my mother's conversations, Bobby had a falling out with my grandfather, and to some degree with Mary Regina. He was estranged from them for long periods of their lives. I thought this might be a result of John's opinionated nature, and family criticism of Bobby's lovely wife Shirley (when she wasn't present) for supposedly being unable to have children. Shirley had to have known about her inability to bear children before she was married, Mary Regina said. I also wondered what John might have thought about his son Bobby being a conscientious objector, if he actually was one.

When Mary Regina was saying things about people that she would not want them to know about, and suddenly realized that I was in the room, she would cut off the conversation and remind the adults: "Walls have ears."

When my uncle Bobby died, Shirley did not inform her in-laws, for some reason unknown to me. We found out about Bobby's death from a nephew's wife. She had Googled Bobby's name and discovered his obituary online.

I liked Bobby and Shirley. I once stumbled upon them kissing in my grandparents' basement when I snuck down there to raid the fruit cellar. Being a kid, I probably went right upstairs and told everybody what I had seen. To my knowledge, Bob and Shirley's marriage lasted till death did them part. Efforts by me to reach Shirley as I wrote this book were unsuccessful.

My grandfather reportedly was able to put away enough during his working days to leave Agnes with sufficient funds and a railroad pension so she could live

Chapter 1: Early Background

without much financial worry until age 92. When Agnes died, in August 1997, reportedly just as her money was running out, she was living in a nice senior living complex.

Her daughter's life was to come to a much different ending.

* * *

Although my Dad eventually would become Mary Regina's next door neighbor, he grew up in another part of town: in Baldwin Township along the City of Pittsburgh's southern border, in a place called Lafferty Hill. I gathered from Mary Regina's occasional derisive remarks that Lafferty Hill was much different from Mary Regina's urban community of Oakland.

Lafferty Hill was a partially rural area when Dad was a child. It was located above the South Pittsburgh waterworks, which processed water from the Monongahela River in open reservoirs for municipal use. When Dad was a child there in the Twenties and Thirties, Lafferty Hill was still growing from its roots as a farming and mining community of the early Nineteen Hundreds. In 1907, for example, Lafferty Elementary School was dedicated as a two-room schoolhouse.

I could not find records describing Lafferty Hill in the Twenties and Thirties, but a June 14, 2000 *Pittsburgh Post-Gazette* article said the area went from "outhouses to septic tanks to sewers" between 1939 and 1957.

I could not imagine my father's family, as I knew them, ever having an outhouse, but I did remember Dad saying that he helped push over a privy during a Halloween prank as a kid. When I raised the subject of an outhouse during a gathering of my cousins for a wedding in 2016,

Chapter 1: Early Background

two cousins recalled hearing a story about one of our aunts accidentally spilling a "thunder bucket" one day as she got ready for a date.

My Dad claimed that his family had been so poor during the Depression that he had to wear his sisters' hand-me-down shoes to school. He had five sisters: three older; Jean, his twin; and one younger. He also had a younger brother. As an adult, Dad would not eat chicken because while living on Lafferty Hill, the family kept chickens and according to Dad chickens were dirty fowl who would eat anything, including cigarette butts and paper milk bottle caps. Dad laughingly recalled that one of the family's chickens had a repulsive cancerous-looking growth on her neck, which he could not forget.

As a boy, my father would roam the paths in Lafferty Hill, high above the Monongahela River, while twin Jean trailed him, looking out for him. "He would throw rocks at me to chase me away. He didn't want me to tattle on him," Jean recalled. "He was a bugger," she commented. Woods remain today in the steep hilly terrain overlooking the river, beyond the area where the Beermans lived.

My father's father (my Grandfather Bill), William Karl Beerman, was born in Plainfield, New Jersey on July 3, 1891 to German American Karl Frederick Wilhelm Beermann, who also was born in New Jersey, and Mary, *nee* Cornelius, Beermann, who was born in the German state of Bahern (Bavaria). My grandfather probably acquired his German accent and some of the language primarily from his mother.

After moving to the Pittsburgh area, Grandfather Bill worked as a nursery keeper, a skilled laborer at Oliver Iron and Steel Company, a drop forge operator in a factory

Chapter 1: Early Background

called Pressed Steel Car, and in his later years, as a night watchman. He and his wife, Catherine, *nee* Bernarding, (my grandmother) successfully raised a large generally happy German Catholic family. During his twenties, Grandfather Bill played banjo in a beer garden band on Pittsburgh's South Side, reportedly much to the disapproval of Catherine. She was born into a Catholic family in Carrick, a neighborhood just inside Pittsburgh's southern border, on March 13, 1895. Catherine was a cousin of Catholic missionary George Elmer Bernarding, former archbishop of Mount Hagan, Papua New Guinea. He also was born in Carrick.

In his older days, Grandfather Bill would sing loudly and unabashedly at some family gatherings, accompanying himself with a guitar or banjo. During such get-togethers, the women, with their children, would fill the living room and dining room, sitting around the table or standing in clusters, all chattering passionately and laughing.

Although Grandfather Bill and his family were religious, he would cuss benignly, without true vulgarity, as he held court in the kitchen with the males, telling jokes in his German accent. He would occasionally spritz out a choice German word, to the delight of his audience members, who seemed to know what the *Deutsch* words meant. They sometimes would laugh so hard that tears ran down their faces. Later, after previewing this book, one of my cousins told me: "Your memory of Grandpap Beerman is spot on. My mother (my Dad's twin Jean) was always shushing him on his profanity. He loved the word bullshit!"

One story told by Grandfather Bill that I remember was about a dog who kept trotting through the narrow walkway between his house and the house next door. The dog would stop to "piss" on his cellar window, and even

Chapter 1: Early Background

into the cellar when the window was open. Grandfather Bill related that one day he waited in ambush down in the cellar with a paint brush full of turpentine. When "the bastard" (the dog) came by and lifted his leg outside the window, Grandfather Bill slapped him in the testicles with the brush, and the "son of a bitch" never pissed there again. Grandfather Bill most likely used the German word *hodensack*, for testicles, in his story.

Grandfather Bill would make his own sauerkraut and beer in his basement, and once entertained a group of visiting relatives with a story about a batch of exploding beer. He said he heard what sounded like -- "BANG .... BANG .... BANG" -- gunshots coming from the cellar, and went down to investigate. He discovered that the rubber bottle stoppers, which had metal pins and wire fasteners attached, had been shot out of his bottles of effervescent homebrew with such force that the "sons of bitches" (pins of the stoppers) imbedded themselves into the floor boards above, which were dripping beer suds.

Despite what the American Society for the Prevention of Cruelty to Animals might think, Grandfather Bill was a kind-hearted, transparent, and loveable man. I recalled visiting him with my father from time to time during the late Sixties after Catherine had died and he was living alone. On Sundays, the widower would dress up in a suit and tie, a black, rich-looking Joseph Horne cashmere overcoat, and a hat, and he would drive to church in his boxy, faded turquoise 1961 or 1962 American Motors Rambler. Presumably he prayed for, or silently conversed with, dearly departed Catherine during Mass.

Grandfather Bill would fake gruffness, but with a hint of humor. Once when Grandfather Bill, my father, and I were having Braunschweiger sandwiches in Grandfather's

Chapter 1: Early Background

kitchen, the canary began singing in his cage near the table, interfering with Grandfather's telling of a story. "Shut up you bastard!" he suddenly snapped at the canary. My reaction was not shock, but projectile laughter -- as I sent a bite of my sandwich flying. His "irascible old man" act was nothing to be afraid of. Grandfather Bill threw the fabric cover over the bird's cage, and remarked in mock disdain, "That was <u>her</u> bird," referring to Catherine. Despite his feigned contempt for the bird, the reality was that he took good care of Catherine's canary after she died, just as he had taken good care of Catherine, who was said to have died while he was holding her in his arms.

While my grandmother Catherine was alive, when my father and I visited her, she would give me some change to buy 15-cent Dell, Marvel, or Classic comic books at the nearby corner store on Grandview Avenue in Mount Washington. When the visit was over and I was leaving with my father, she would give me a "*kuss*," German for kiss, and a "poke" (small brown paper bag) containing an orange or an apple, or she would put one or two coins into my hand. "Don't tell your father," she would whisper.

I told Grandfather Bill about my job at the *New Pittsburgh Courier* one day. It was during a visit I made alone to see my widower grandfather in 1970. The *Courier* office was nearby on Carson Street, and I was sneaking a break from work, delaying my return to the office after an assignment. The scene was grandfather and grandson sitting on the front porch during a summer afternoon. I observed that unlike Grandfather John, Grandfather Bill had no nasty comment to make about n-----s upon hearing that his grandson was working for a black newspaper. I felt that Grandfather Bill respected me, even though I was just a kid, barely 21 years old.

Chapter 1: Early Background

That was the year before Grandfather Bill died after a short illness. While he was hospitalized, my Dad and I visited him in his room at South Side Hospital. As he lay in his hospital bed, Grandfather Bill told his son and grandson that he could imagine that his heart was bleeding inside his chest, like those pictures of the Sacred Heart on holy cards.

When I learned that Grandfather Bill had died, I had one of my life's stronger spiritual experiences. "Such a soul as his could not simply die and disappear," I thought. "He must still exist somewhere and there must be an afterlife."

After Grandfather Bill died, in February 1971 at the age of 80, I informally inherited his black Joseph Horne overcoat and I wore it to work on cold winter days for decades. I would sometimes think of my grandfather as I was leaving for work, when I took his coat out of the closet to put it on. My Dad's siblings bestowed upon him their father's old Rambler car, since Dad was suffering hard financial times as he went through his long divorce litigation. It was the best car Dad had for a while, until a control arm failed and caused a front wheel to break off.

* * *

In August 1943 the Beermans bought their frame house at 305 Kathleen Street in the ethnic German Mount Washington section of the City of Pittsburgh, where my grandparents would live out the remainder of their lives. The family home came to be known as "up on the hill," because not only was it on Mount Washington, but Kathleen Street itself was hilly, and the houses on the Beermans' side of the street had long sets of concrete steps ascending to them, with handrails fashioned from threaded galvanized pipe and couplings.

Chapter 1: Early Background

Grandfather Bill kept the house in fine condition. Down in his cellar, he mixed his own paint with linseed oil, and his cream-and-black colored paint job on the wooden front porch balustrades and columns made them look like ivory and ebony. Even the stairs to his attic shined, with blue-gray glossy paint. Grandfather Bill had gardens in his back yard. He fitted them with glass frames to protect them from frost in spring and fall. There were screens to keep the birds off the lettuce and other vegetables in the summer. He enhanced the soil in his garden with ashes from a 55-gallon ash barrel that he kept at the far edge of his yard.

Years after Grandfather Bill died and the house had been sold, it burned down and now there is a gap in the row of homes on Kathleen Street where the Beermans once dwelled. Learning of the fire reminded me that once after the holidays my grandfather disposed of the branches of his Christmas tree in his living room fireplace, which had a very strong draft. The ferocity of the roaring blaze that ensued seemed to threaten the house, and scared everyone watching. I wondered whether that living room fireplace had played a role in the fire that destroyed the house decades later.

***

During my youth, the Beermans were a family who would gather around the piano to sing. My father had a voice like Bing Crosby. As an adult, I won a Christmas carol trivia contest at an office party because I knew more of the lyrics of the songs than anyone else. I attributed my exceptional memory for the lyrics of carols to the Christmas season gatherings up on the hill.

Chapter 1: Early Background

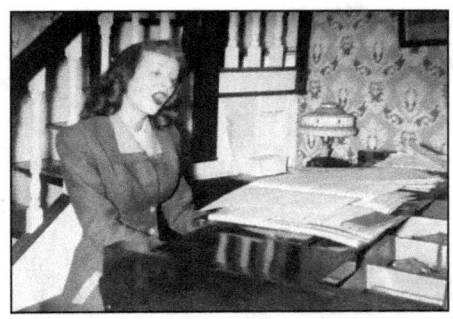

My Aunt Ruth at the piano "up on the hill" in the late 1940s.

On Christmas Eve someone would dim the lights and my Dad's twin Jean, who wore the Santa suit even though she was quite petite, would spread cheer. She would pass out gifts from a white cloth sack, and give each of the many grandchildren in attendance some individual attention.

Any time the generations convened for a holiday or birthday celebration up on the hill, good spirits, conversation, and laughter would flood the house. The Beerman girls were amazingly fluent. The words flowed from them freely like water down a stream, and each girl was skilled at breaking in to add her contribution to the conversation, which was nonstop merriment. It was as if everyone was high on marijuana or speeding on amphetamines, which, of course, they were not. They didn't even drink much, and I remember that I thought it was odd when I once saw one of my aunts with a brown bottle of beer. Aunt Ruth became in my memories "the one who drinks beer."

Two of the girls, Ruth and Ede, married Greyhound bus drivers, both of whom told lots of funny stories; many of the anecdotes were about bus passengers or motorists. One of the bus drivers, Ede's husband Benedict M. Duffner, smoked big cigars and reminded me of comedian George Burns. Two of the girls, Sis and Honey, married engineers, one of whom reportedly oversaw construction of

Chapter 1: Early Background

a steel mill in South Africa. Jean married a car inspector for P&LE Railroad. Dad's younger brother Bob became a switchman for Bell Telephone. All of the seven siblings and their spouses and children would show up for some special occasions up on the hill and the families would pack the house.

During the year 2016, almost 50 years after I had last seen Uncle Ben Duffner, I received a check out of the blue from Ben's estate. The Greyhound driver's bequests totaled more than $750,000. Ben left much of his money to Father Flanagan's Boys Town, in Omaha, NE; Auberle Home for Boys (the Boys Town of the East) in McKeesport, PA; two Catholic churches; and a Catholic monastery.

Getting the check from someone whose name I had not heard in nearly a half century caused me to experience detailed flashbacks. I began to remember the individual facial expressions, voices, and personalities of the relatives who had been at those family gatherings up on the hill, not just the overview scenes of the group as a whole. Also, I was reminded of how the Catholic faith was infused throughout the family. My relatives were very good people, I realized. I spiritually thanked Ben Duffner for reminding me of my heritage by sending the check from the beyond.

I remember riding with my father through the snow-covered streets of Mount Oliver toward Mount Washington on the way to one of the Beermans' Christmas Eve gatherings up on the hill. It was like driving through a moonlit, urban-neighborhood winter wonderland scene from an old black-and-white movie, except that the homes lining the streets had colored Christmas lights -- the old-fashioned kind with big bulbs -- with halos around them from the moisture in the cold air. I recalled seeing in the headlights the tire tracks of only one or two automobiles in

Chapter 1: Early Background

the snow ahead on the cobblestone streets, and the gleaming steel streetcar rails. It was a nearly silent night, as the snow absorbed most of the sounds made by the car.

Mary Regina did not especially like to go up on the hill, for a reason I never determined. I wondered if she often skipped the gatherings at the Beermans' because she had said something that she was embarrassed about, and was uncomfortable with her in-laws. Mary Regina was the only girl in her childhood home, while there were five Beerman sisters. Maybe she felt outnumbered. Or maybe she was sulking or moping after arguments with my father or she simply was sick and did not feel like going to parties. Or maybe she felt the gifts being taken for the kids at a party were inadequate because my father was laid off and money was tight. Whatever the reason, Mary Regina would avoid the visits up on the hill, and they became bonding experiences for my father and me.

***

My father withdrew from Baldwin High School, where he was a vocational student, during his sophomore year on March 21, 1942, just weeks after turning age 17. At the time, his transcript showed five Ds and three Cs for ninth grade and five Ds for part of his tenth. His record contained no entry for an IQ score; he probably missed the test. Grandfather Bill's occupation at the time was listed on my Dad's school record as a "florist" at a greenhouse in the Pittsburgh city neighborhood of Carrick. The family address was recorded as 782 Agnew Road, one of at least two places where the Beermans had lived on Lafferty Hill. My father's Baldwin High School record showed Code G as the reason for withdrawal. Code G was defined as "Legally Employed. Employment Certificate." Obtaining

Chapter 1: Early Background

the certificate was commonly referred to as "getting your working papers."

My father possibly left school to help my grandfather in his work as a greenhouse keeper and earn some income for the family. Dad once told me that he did not like working at the greenhouse for "the old man," which is what he called his father, because the clay flower pots were heavy and the work was hard.

An Army enlistment civilian-occupation record shows Dad also worked spray painting the inside and outside of "shells" at the Pittsburgh Water Heater Company for 10 months after quitting school and before entering the Army. I wondered whether the "shells" were water heater shells (tanks) or whether the company converted from making water heaters to making large rounds for naval guns for the war.

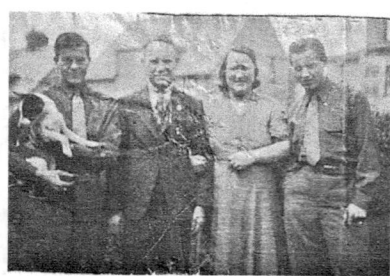

Dad, right, in Swansea in 1944 with another soldier and hosts Reginald John Peachey and his wife Dorothy Clarissa May Peachey, and the Peachey family dog, Bett.

Dad's family moved to Kathleen Street up on the hill the summer after he was inducted into the Army at age 18, on May 12, 1943.

Dad sailed for Wales on December 29, 1943 and was recorded as being in Swansea, Wales on January 11, 1944. He was billeted with a family named Peachey. He stayed at 62 Dyfed Ave, in the Townhill section, with the Peacheys -- Reginald John, a press tool setter for a metal box company, his wife, Dorothy Clarissa May Peachey, three children, and a dog named Bett -- for about 6 months.

Chapter 1: Early Background

After the Normandy invasion in June, 1944, Dad was shipped off to France where he was a crane operator, private first class, possibly with General George Patton's Third Army, or with the Seventh Army. Dad told me that he helped pull sunken vessels out of harbors, and loaded and unloaded trucks and railroad cars. It was a great adventure for him and he would later reminisce about eating sun-warmed aromatic cantaloupes from a farmer's field along a road in the French countryside between Normandy and Paris, and later visiting a Paris nightclub that had a raunchy stage show featuring a woman and a horse.

Dad's military records were sketchy because most were lost in a fire on July 12, 1973 at the National Personnel Records Center archives in St. Louis, along with millions of other records of Army and Air Corps/Air Force servicemen. The surviving four pages of his records documented that he served in the Northern France, Southern France, and Rhineland Campaigns. I have vague memories of Dad's army jacket hanging in a closet when I was a kid. I remember seeing a shoulder patch with the letter "A" on the jacket. Patton's Third Army had a patch with an "A" inside a circle, and the Seventh Army had a patch that itself was shaped like a wide triangular "A."

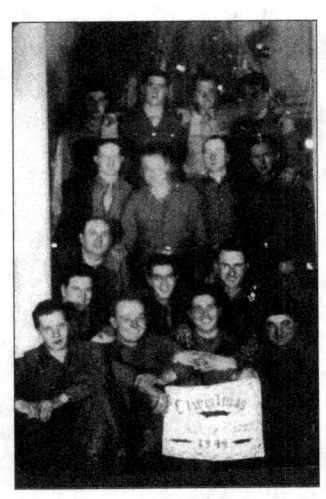

Dad, lower left, "over there," in France, on Christmas, 1944

For 15 years or so after the war the Peacheys would occasionally mail letters and gifts to Dad and his family. I remember blue and red airmail envelopes and stamps depicting Queen Elizabeth, and packages arriving with knitted sweaters and Cadbury chocolates. I especially prized a thick wool cable-knit tennis sweater sent for me.

In 2015 I got in touch with some Peachey family descendants. I located them with help from *South Wales Evening Post* senior reporter Geraint Thomas, who printed a story about my Dad and the Peacheys. Swansea librarian Claire Tranter and archivist David Morris were also helpful.

A niece of the Peacheys, Miss Dorothea Hilda Peachey, was on her deathbed in a hospital when she learned of my search for Peachey family members. Before she died on June 5, 2015 at age 86, she asked a friend, Mrs. Jean Guest, to email me and help with my research. Miss Peachey enjoyed helping people. She was a religious person who volunteered even while an octogenarian as a "street pastor" standing by in a downtown church, St. David's, from 10 p.m. until 4 a.m., praying to assist anyone in need of help at night in Swansea City. "The stories of her generosity and kindness are legion," said her eulogist Alan McNally.

I was able to talk with John Peachey, son of Reginald John and Dorothy, who recognized his dog as well as his parents in a photo of Dad with the Peacheys. However, John was only 4-1/2 at the time the photo was taken, and could remember only that his family took in American GIs. John Peachey most likely was the last person alive in Wales who knew anything at all about my father.

I once saw tears well up in Dad's eyes while he watched a re-run of the 1942 movie, *Yankee Doodle Dandy*, as actor James Cagney, playing entertainer George

Chapter 1: Early Background

M. Cohan, sang the stirring patriotic song, *Over There*, while marching in an on-screen parade of American soldiers going off to war. The song, which Cohan wrote in 1917 when the U.S. entered World War I, goes in part:

> *Over there, over there*
> *Send the word, send the word, over there*
> *That the Yanks are coming*
> *The Yanks are coming...over there.*

The movie is said to have inspired many young Americans to enlist for World War II. When the movie was released on June 6, 1942, Dad was 17. I do not know whether my father enlisted or was drafted, but his tears seemed to reveal a quiet patriotism and secret pride in his military service. After seeing my father tear up, I do it too when I hear the song.

Dad earned the honor due a soldier who went to war. But postwar when people asked the common question, "What did you do in the war?" as far as I knew, Dad's answer lacked the prestige of that of a combat veteran such as a 101st Airborne soldier who suffered in the Battle of the Bulge, or a Marine who fought through the horrors in the Pacific. When, as a kid, I asked Dad if he ever had been shot at, he told me he once had to dive down some steps along a sidewalk in Paris because a sniper was shooting at him. He must have gotten to Paris just as the Germans were evacuating. That was the extent of what the father told the son about the "action" he saw in the war.

A famous photo shows Parisians coming under sniper fire while celebrating the liberation. A caption for the photo states: "Crowds of Parisians celebrating the entry of Allied troops into Paris scatter for cover as a sniper fires from a building on the *Place de la Concorde*. Although the

Chapter 1: Early Background

Germans surrendered the city, small bands of snipers still remained. 08/26/1944." (National Archives Identifier 531206.) A MOVIETONE NEWS newsreel video of the Liberation and Paris sniper attacks, with commentator Lowell Thomas, is at https://www.youtube.com/watch?v=_wiEJoGcCg8. (footage farm 22 04 69)

I gained a deeper appreciation of my father's service from the book, "*G.I. Limey,*" written by Geraint Thomas about Clifford Guard, a Welsh immigrant to America who enlisted in the U.S. Army and fought through France with the 3rd Armored Division, known as the Spearhead Division. Guard passed through the Fort Indiantown Gap, Pennsylvania staging area 4 months before my Dad did. Just like Dad, he sailed across the Atlantic to England on a troop ship, stayed in the U.K. until June 1944, sailed across the English Channel to France, spent the rest of 1944 and part of 1945 in France, and redeployed to the U.S. through Nice, the largest city on the French Riviera.

Guard's detailed eyewitness accounts and comments in his book make it clear that while Guard was at the perilous leading edge of warfare, many soldiers elsewhere in France in 1944 or 1945, with nominally noncombat duties, were also in danger and were lucky to get home alive. He wrote, for example, that Normandy remained somewhat dangerous for weeks after D-Day.

Later in life, when he was older, Dad would demonstrate that although he was small in stature and had a quiet disposition, he had the substance necessary to help build the nation and contribute to the reputation of the Greatest Generation. He overcame limiting adversities and put together a successful civilian career, in which he directed more than 100 steelworkers, many of them very

Chapter 1: Early Background

manly veterans, as a foreman in the challenging environment of a steel mill.

***

While Dad was overseas, as fate would have it, the Beermans got to know their new next-door neighbors, the Fishers, who lived then at 303 Kathleen Street. The stage was set for a storybook romance when the war ended and Dad came home.

During the war, Mary Regina Fisher became friends with her neighbor, Jean Beerman, Dad's twin sister. Both were pretty girls sharing the nickname Jean -- one formally Regina and the other Eugenia -- and they both got jobs in downtown Pittsburgh. Mary Regina Fisher joined the Reliance Life Insurance Company of Pittsburgh in the Dividend Accounting Department, beginning in the summer of 1943. Jean Beerman became a legal secretary in the politically connected P.J. McArdle law firm at about the same time. P.J. McArdle was a Pittsburgh city councilman and the namesake of the P.J. McArdle Roadway, which angles up the north side of Mount Washington. His son, Joseph A., became a Pittsburgh city councilman and a U.S. congressman.

Each weekday morning, on their way to work together, the two Jeans would ride the Monongahela Incline down the side of Mount Washington to Carson Street, along what is now the Station Square district. Then they would use the Smithfield Street Bridge to walk over the Monongahela River into town.

So it seemed natural that Dad, the returning GI who was the twin of Mary Regina's friend, and Mary Regina, the girl next door, would date and fall in love.

Chapter 1: Early Background

Jean (Eugenia) Beerman would remain close to me her entire life. She was the last girl to leave the nest on Kathleen Street to marry. Before that, while still at home, she was selected -- for the most appropriate reasons -- as my godmother. I remember visits up on the hill when my godmother, then a lovely girl in her twenties, would sit and talk with me in her enchanting, husky voice. She would sometimes tell me about Jesus, and I remember her giving me a rosary. I was Jean's twin brother's little boy, and she would serve as my second mother throughout my life. Aunt Jean and her eventual family of six children -- my cousins -- would treat me better and show me more affection than anyone else, except for my father, my grandmother, Agnes, and, sometimes, my Mexican-American second wife of more than 26 years, Martha Del Avellano Beerman, and my children.

Eventually, when my godmother met my wife Martha, they bonded immediately. Both being loquacious, they chattered away in a wide-ranging conversation. Part of it was about their favorite Catholic saints. Jean gave Martha a bracelet with religious icons on it. Jean later privately advised me that Martha was "a keeper." My godmother's opinion of Martha carried such weight with me that remembering it helped me get through the times of uncertainty in my marriage.

Six decades after my early visits with my godmother up on the hill, I would give the eulogies for both my mother and my godmother in 2011 and 2013 respectively. My godmother and her daughter Kathy accompanied me in the funeral car and provided me with much appreciated support as I handled my mother's funeral arrangements in 2011. I am proud that I share some of my godmother's genes,

Chapter 1: Early Background

which I believe account for much of whatever goodness I possess.

Godmother Jean spent her adult life married to 6-foot-2 Fred Smith, a very pleasant former amateur baseball player who seemed always to be relaxed and smiling calmly as he told interesting stories about people he had known. The couple reminded me of Jimmy Stewart and June Allyson in the movie, *The Stratton Story*, although Jean looked more like Jane Fonda than June Allyson, and Jean had a more outgoing personality than Allyson. *The Stratton Story*, a 1949 movie about a real-life major league pitcher, was billed as "One of the great love stories of our time."

For almost 4 decades, Jean would attend Mass every business day at lunchtime at St. Mary of Mercy Church, at Stanwix Street and Boulevard of the Allies, near her office. For many years, into their seventies, Jean and Fred delivered Meals On Wheels to homebound people in their town of Castle Shannon, PA. In 2016, after the deaths of Jean and Fred, some of their children and grandchildren helped host a Thanksgiving Day sit-down lunch for the homeless at St. Mary of Mercy.

As far as I could tell, the entire Smith family led essentially happy lives and Jean and Fred's six children collectively took excellent care of them in their old age.

The Smiths led me to notice that it seemed many of the nicer people I knew tended to be religious, and that people from large families tended to seem happier. This also appeared true for my cousins on the Fisher side, all of whom seemed to be good people. The Fishers helped my mother out during her old age and illnesses. They also helped me ready her apartment for a new tenant and

Chapter 1: Early Background

dispose of her things after her death. The Smiths and the Fishers were conscious of the needs of others, and would do whatever they could for people.

On Memorial Day in 2015, one of Jean Smith's adult children, my cousin Lisa Tharp, posted on Facebook a photo of the gravestone of Jean and Fred. Upon seeing the picture of the memorial with the names of my uncle and aunt, a thought occurred to me: "Surely this is one couple who truly are 'resting in peace' together. Their time on earth was well spent."

Sadly, the lives of Jean Smith's twin, my Dad, and his wife Mary Regina, my mother, would be tragically different.

***

My Dad was said to have had "looks," just as Mary Regina did, when they met, and Mary Regina was impressed that he always wore white shirts, which he ironed himself. I thought that photos from their dating days -- the usual poses with drinks at a bistro table -- resembled Hollywood publicity shots.

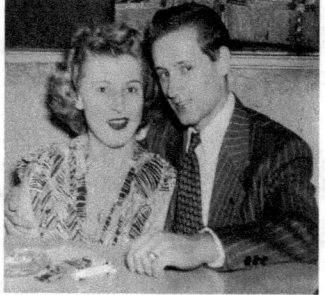

Mary Regina and Dad in August 1946

When the storybook marriage was failing, Mary Regina would complain that she had been fooled by Dad's white shirts, which were not part of his normal attire later when he was a steel worker (when he had grease under his blackened and split fingernails and scraped knuckles), and that her marriage to him had destroyed her own "looks" and health. Ironically, Mary Regina's hatred and vendetta-like

Chapter 1: Early Background

torture of Dad while she waged a brutal war of divorce eventually helped drive him to an early death at age 64, but she lived on for 22 more years.

The divorce even tore apart the two Jeans, who had shared the name Jean Beerman for a few years after Mary Regina's marriage to Dad and before Eugenia's marriage to Fred Smith. Dad's twin took his side in the divorce conflict, and she arranged for her law firm to represent Dad in the legal battle. Jean Smith and her family also came to Dad's rescue during the dark days of loneliness after his marriage broke up, allowing him to hang out at their home, and he very much enjoyed the company of his nieces and nephews.

Before they died, though, while they were in their eighties, the two Jeans reconciled, both being at that time God-fearing Catholics.

Chapter 2: Marriage and a Family

On May 21, 1947, about 20 months after Dad's discharge from the Army, Mary Regina and Dad wed at St. George's Catholic Church in Carrick. The wedding party included a friend of Dad's, who is not identified here, his friend's wife (who Mary Regina would later name in a divorce allegation), Dad's twin, Jean, his brother Bob, and Mary Regina's brother, Jack.

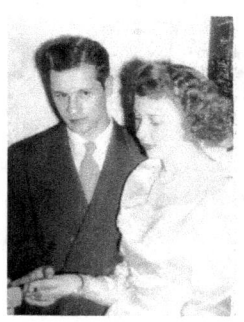

Cutting the cake on the first day of the marriage from hell.

A lifetime later during the funeral Mass for Dad's twin Jean at an old Catholic church in Carrick, I would gaze at the altar and envision that in a different slice of time my parents had stood at such an altar in Carrick to be married, blissfully unaware of the horrible fates awaiting them.

The wedding reception was at Mary Regina's house on Kathleen Street, next door to Dad's house. I think the newlyweds honeymooned in Washington, D.C. I wasn't

Chapter 2: Marriage and a Family

sure, but I thought I'd heard that they took a Greyhound bus.

Almost 2 decades after the wedding, Mary Regina would complain in a divorce document that after their honeymoon, the couple had to move in with her parents for 2 or 3 weeks because Dad had been laid off from work.

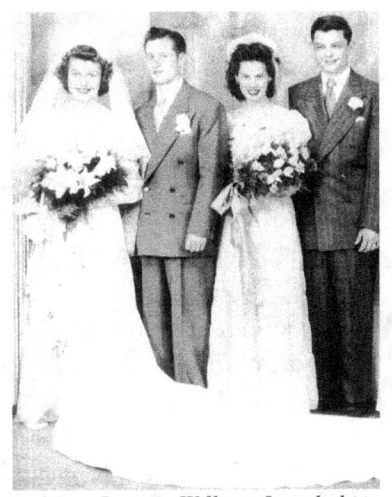

Mary Regina, William Joseph, his twin Jean, and Mary Regina's brother Jack

Dad worked for a time after the war as a redcap for Greyhound Bus Company at its terminal in downtown Pittsburgh. After Greyhound, he applied his Army experience and skill as a crane operator in a civilian job for "J&L," the Jones and Laughlin Steel Company. He became a craneman in J&L's mill between Second Avenue and the Monongahela River's northern shoreline in Pittsburgh.

Dad and Mary Regina rented an apartment for a while from Dad's aforementioned friend, at 521 Agnew Road, Lafferty Hill, three blocks from where Dad lived while he was in high school. Agnew Road ran from Becks Run Road, past the South Pittsburgh Water Works, and up into Lafferty Hill. They were living there when I was born in October 1948. Mary Regina alleged that while they resided at 521 Agnew, events occurred that she would bring up repeatedly as the years went by. As a child, I heard vague references to the claimed occurrences. I later surmised that

Chapter 2: Marriage and a Family

possibly, in Mary Regina's mind, Dad had engaged in misconduct, real or imagined, with some other woman, possibly his friend's wife.

After my parents had moved into their own home, and I was about 5 or 6 years old, my father took me on a junk-hunting trip along some back roads in his old neighborhood of Lafferty Hill. On the way, we stopped at a gas station that Dad called Dave's on Becks Run Road, where Dad bought me a bottle of pop and a pack of Lance peanut butter crackers from a big glass display jar on Dave's counter. It was a quaint gas station, even for the Fifties. It had greenish-gray motor oil for sale in clear glass quart jars with screw-on metal spouts, and the driveway to the pumps was unpaved.

After Dad spent some time talking with Dave, an elderly man whom Dad apparently knew well, the father and his son drove off to look for lifeless console radios among the junk that people had thrown out at dumping grounds along dirt roads. Television had just come out, which might explain the easy availability of radios at the dumps. Dad could resurrect dead radios and he picked up some nice specimens including models with cat's-eye blue lights whose pupils would narrow to indicate that a broadcast was tuned in optimally. Some radios would pick up short-wave bands and ship-to-shore Morse code. Today they would be prized antiques.

On this particular father-son radio-hunting trip, Dad stopped along the road to talk through the car window with a woman he knew. When I mentioned the stop later at home, Mary Regina became furious. This was an early sign of how the marriage would end badly.

Chapter 2: Marriage and a Family

I wondered as I worked on this book after Mary Regina's death whether Dad might have told me to wait in the car while he ducked into the woman's house. If I had told such a thing to my mother, her reaction would have been understandable. But as an adult I could not remember exactly what happened or what I had told my mother.

Later Mary Regina would repeatedly accuse Dad of vague improper conduct with various neighbors and even with a woman who was well known to my elementary school classmates. Mary Regina said in a court document that she and my father quarreled every 2 months or so about other women.

That my father was involved with the "well known woman" or neighbor women seemed to me to be bizarre and incredible ideas. Although I could never be sure, based on my observations as I grew up, I did not think Mary Regina had credibility or competent situational awareness.

I began to have sympathy for my father and I took a liking to him much as a pet dog bonds with a certain member of a household for some reason. I noticed as an adult that my own dogs, Lobo, a bright German shepherd, and Moose, a dim but lovable pit bull, would get up and leave the room if I raised my voice toward my wife Martha. The dogs obviously perceived me to be the aggressor, and they liked Martha better. Yet, dogs did not understand the substance of the arguments. For what it was worth, I sympathized with my Dad.

After writing about my memories, I became concerned that I might be remembering my family life as a youth inaccurately, and that my impressions from my boyhood were imagined, prejudiced against my mother, or exaggerated. So, when I was 66 years old, researching my book, I obtained from the Allegheny County Courthouse some half-century-old records from my parents' divorce case. The records reassured me that my memories were accurate, in essence. I was relieved. If I had seen things incorrectly, then so had the court, and we both were wrong. Mary Regina might have been right all along, but it just didn't seem that way.

Most of the court records from 13 years of divorce litigation were missing ("Not in the box," as court official Michael R. Murphy said after a thorough search that extended over a couple of weeks), but one retrieved record was a revealing report by a divorce hearing officer called a master. Masters were lawyers who presided over divorce trials in place of judges, and they made recommendations to a designated judge in each case. The master in the Beerman case, Daniel T. Zamos, Esq., heard on March 14, 1969 a full day of testimony in the first trial in Mary Regina's suit for divorce.

I noted that the "well known woman" and her husband, who lived near us, had been brought to the Allegheny County Courthouse in downtown Pittsburgh to testify. The situation was mortifying. The woman denied ever being alone with Dad. Her husband expressed faith in his wife and said she would have had no opportunity for a rendezvous with Dad.

In his report to the judge, the master summarized Mary Regina's testimony from both direct and cross examinations. He commented, "The plaintiff obviously was a high-strung, highly nervous individual who suffered some sort of physical affliction which was not fully determined." He wrote that she showed "extreme jealousy," and that, "The incidents related by her concerning other women were trivial, at best, and would hardly have affected the sensibilities of the average wife." The master concluded that she had failed to prove she was entitled to a divorce. The report, along with Mary Regina's Bill of Particulars, or allegations, depicted to me a pathetic performance by my mother. The hearing master formally recommended that Mary Regina's petition for a divorce be denied.

If the divorce case, which ultimately continued for a total of 4,900 days, truly did stem from "trivial" matters, as the master said, then what it did to the couple and their family was all the more tragic.

In her court filings, Mary Regina accused Dad of aggravating her health problems, which included Addison's disease, an abnormality of the adrenal gland, by deliberately causing Mary Regina stress. I looked up Addison's disease, and found that its symptoms could include depression, anxiety, and changes in personality. In extreme cases, it could result in psychosis, or delusions -- false beliefs that a person holds on to without adequate evidence. Since Mary Regina also had thyroid disease, which can cause fatigue and depression, I thought that the dynamic interaction of thyroid disease and Addison's disease could have affected my mother to a severe or even an extreme degree.

In addition to pain in her marriage inflicted by haunting jealousy, which reminded me of the Elvis Presley songs, *"Suspicion,"* and *"Suspicious Minds,"* Mary Regina probably was experiencing culture shock and depression caused by her surroundings.

* * *

Mom and Dad moved from Lafferty Hill to Port Vue, Pennsylvania, in 1950, after Dad got a job as a craneman at

Chapter 2: Marriage and a Family

National Tube Works, a steel mill complex owned by U.S. Steel Corporation in nearby McKeesport. The City of McKeesport lies among smaller towns in the Monongahela Valley, which has been called the "Steel Valley" and the "Cradle of the Steel Industry." National Tube itself once employed 10,000.

Both Lafferty Hill and Port Vue were much different from Oakland, the cultural center of Pittsburgh, where Mary Regina grew up.

In relocating to Port Vue, Mary Regina, a girl from Andrew Carnegie's cultural enclave in Oakland, moved to one of Carnegie's mill towns.

Mary Regina's parents, meanwhile, moved to a Roman brick twin on a tree-lined street in Dormont, a pleasant borough sharing borders with the City of Pittsburgh and Mount Lebanon Township, where many of Pittsburgh's Fortune 500 corporate executives lived during the Fifties and Sixties.

The Beerman family -- Dad, Mary Regina, and I -- would drive to Dormont from Port Vue almost every Sunday to spend the day with the Fishers. In those days Dormont was an example of America at near its lower-middle-class nicest. It had streetcar service to downtown Pittsburgh, which was only 5 or 10 minutes away, and it had its own thriving main street business district – West Liberty Avenue. Homes in Dormont were affordable, costing a fraction of the value of mansions in neighboring Mount Lebanon, but Dormont nevertheless had a very pleasant ambiance. Dormont was known for having the best Fourth of July fireworks in Allegheny County, and possibly the best public swimming pool. Dormont pool, at 60,000

Chapter 2: Marriage and a Family

square feet, was one of the largest in Pennsylvania and it was declared an historic landmark.

On Tolma Avenue, where the Fishers lived, even the bricks in the pavement of the street were clean. The homes and their small front yards were as neat as could be. Large maple trees lining the sidewalks kept the Fishers' front porch cool in the summer. The trees seemed to freshen the air with the oxygen they generated. The leaves were shiny and a deep green in color, with the veins distinctly visible, and they were free of the particulate pollution dust that accumulated on everything in parts of the Steel Valley.

The Fishers' porch was the perfect place for the adults to converse or read the Sunday newspaper. One of the two porch gliders offered a comfortable spot for a kid to take a nap, even in July in the afternoon while the locusts were singing noisily in the trees.

John Fisher belonged to a Catholic church named St. Bernard's, which was located on the Dormont-Mount Lebanon line. St. Bernard's was magnificent. When I later saw the National Cathedral in Washington, DC, it reminded me of St. Bernard's, although the cathedral has three towers and St. Bernard's has only one.

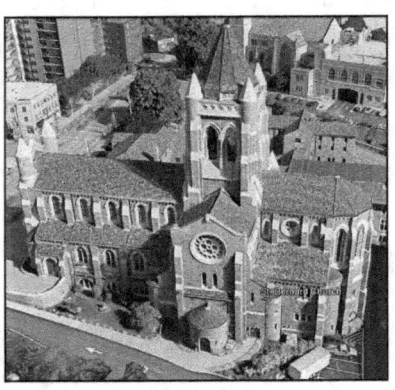

St. Bernard's Church Google Earth

In contrast to St. Bernard's and St. Paul's Cathedral parish, where Mary Regina went to high school, her humble parish in Port Vue, St Joseph's, had a church in the

Chapter 2: Marriage and a Family

basement of the single-story St. Joseph's elementary school, which I would eventually attend.

Although Mary Regina would go to Mass each morning in her old age while living in a senior citizen apartment building managed by a nun, during my time with her, she rarely attended Mass at our local parish church, St. Joseph's. She would send me to Sunday Mass to put the donation envelopes into the collection basket, probably hoping the Polish Felician sisters who staffed the school would not realize she didn't go to church. She unfailingly would ask me for the "church paper" (bulletin) when I returned from church, most likely to obtain some assurance that I had not skipped, and to verify that the Beermans' donation envelopes were listed in the bulletin among the previous Sunday's contributions. Mary Regina said she didn't attend St. Joseph's because of her ill health and diminished "looks," and because the pastor berated the parishioners in his sermons for not giving enough money to the church, "although he rides around in his big black Chrysler."

Mom and Dad bought their Port Vue house in a new development of low-cost starter homes called Westwood Hills. The development was built to take advantage of the government-guaranteed GI Bill financing for such homes for the servicemen who were marrying after returning from the war. The developer bought hilly farmland and put in streets and hundreds of Cape Cod cookie-cutter houses built with asbestos shingle siding.

Their house had a combination living room-dining room; a kitchen; a utility room with a wringer washer, electric dryer, water heater, and forced air furnace; a bathroom; and two bedrooms, all on one floor. The house

Chapter 2: Marriage and a Family

had steel-framed single-pane crank-out windows that sweated or iced up depending on the weather, and Mary Regina had to put towels on the window sills to soak up the water from condensation or melting ice. The floor was a concrete slab with dark-brown 9-inch-square vinyl-asbestos tiles pasted on it with mastic. Imbedded in the slab when the concrete was poured were return ducts for the forced-air furnace.

The original pre-war town of Port Vue was tree-canopied and it had brick homes concentrated along Romine Avenue and connecting streets. At an elevation of 945 feet, it overlooked the City of McKeesport, which stands at the confluence of the Monongahela and Youghiogheny Rivers; hence the name Port Vue. The new modest frame homes were built higher up on the hills above the original older community. The Beermans' home was near the top of the borough, at elevation 1,140 feet.

Contrary to what the town's name implied, the view from Port Vue was not a feature to brag about, especially at night. Most of the GI homes did not even have views. Our home did, but the view was not of McKeesport to the east. During the day, we could see to the northwest for miles through our egg-crate style front "picture window." We could watch planes coming in for landings at the Allegheny County Airport on a plateau across the Monongahela River Valley in West Mifflin. Also, we could see storms approaching long before they arrived. Winds blew forcefully across the hilltop.

But the view at night in the McKeesport area in the Fifties and Sixties sometimes resembled James Parton's famous description of Pittsburgh a century earlier in 1868: "Hell with the lid off." Tall, roiling plumes of blue, yellow, and orange flame jetted out of the stacks at the mill, which

Chapter 2: Marriage and a Family

was located between the Monongahela River and McKeesport's main thoroughfare, Lyle Boulevard. Smoke, steam, and sulfuric acid mist rose from the Coke Works, across the Monongahela River in Clairton. And fire and smoke spewed from the furnaces at the U.S. Steel works in nearby Duquesne.

Dad told me that the mills purposely blew out their dirtiest smoke at night, when it was less noticeable. The particulate fallout was everywhere downwind, and winter snowfalls did not leave the landscape looking snow-white for long. Rather, a day after the snow stopped, dust was visible on the surface of the snow, or the snow turned to dirty gray slush, frozen or soft, depending on the temperature.

The area was part of the dreary setting for the Robert De Niro movie *Deer Hunter*. Particularly, sections of Clairton, Duquesne, and McKeesport provided a cultural and visual backdrop for *Deer Hunter*. When I first saw the 1978 movie, I immediately recognized part of my childhood environment. The town in the movie was a composite of steel towns in Pennsylvania, Ohio, and elsewhere. Clairton, said to be the primary setting for the movie, was more of a depressed town than McKeesport or Port Vue, in my memory. But many towns in the Steel Valley shared certain typical environmental characteristics like those depicted in the movie.

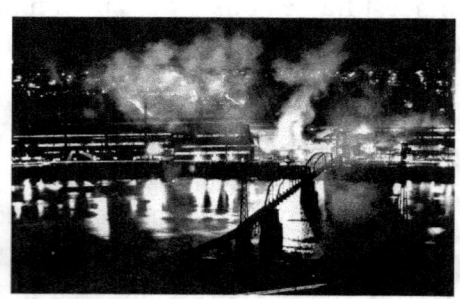

U.S. Steel National Works in McKeesport circa 1950.
Photo: Carnegie Library of Pittsburgh, Pa. Dept.

Chapter 2: Marriage and a Family

Although the night sky over Port Vue and the surrounding area was often orange, not black, the nights there eerily seemed to be extremely dark at ground level, visually, and psychologically. On foggy nights and mornings, the air in Port Vue was sometimes gray, and sometimes yellowish brown, probably from sulfur and rust molecules in the air. Once, shortly after Dad painted our house buttercup yellow, a fog turned the house yellowish brown. Fortunately, acid rain and Dad's efforts with a garden hose and a scrub brush washed off the brown film.

One day, Dad took me to get a car part at an automobile junk yard located outside of the City of Glassport, which adjoined Port Vue on the east side of the Monongahela River across from the Clairton coke works. I found that I could poke my index finger through hoods and fenders of some of the cars in the yard. I assumed this was because they had been rusted and corroded by sulfuric acid in the air.

People driving along River Road across the river from the coke works could sometimes see pinhead-size, probably acidic, droplets appear on their windshields even during dry weather. The side of the hill on the Glassport side of the Monongahela River, across from the coke ovens, was barren of live vegetation, and had remnants of spooky-looking dead trees like those in war movie scenes showing the aftermath of heavy shelling of a wooded battlefield. From my environment, I learned long before today's environmentalists about acid rain.

The Steel Valley world 13 miles south of Mary Regina's parents' home in lovely Dormont was not all bad, though. The people were the best. I remember my grade school classmates with fondness. Nowhere could a congregation sing hymns more beautifully and fervently

Chapter 2: Marriage and a Family

than my good neighbors and classmates in that basement church in Port Vue. And I never witnessed a more moving scene than the grade school girls in their blue dresses singing *Immaculate Mary, our hearts are on fire,"* in the May Queen procession around the school grounds, with the scent of spring blossoms in the air. *"Ave, Ave, Ave Maria,"* they sang, and then, *Oh Holy Queen enthroned above . . . . S-al-ve, s-al-ve, s-al-ve, Re-gin-a.*

Regarding the environment, there were pretty scenes as well as eyesores. There were trees and gardens, and impressive residential and commercial architecture in the older parts of the area.

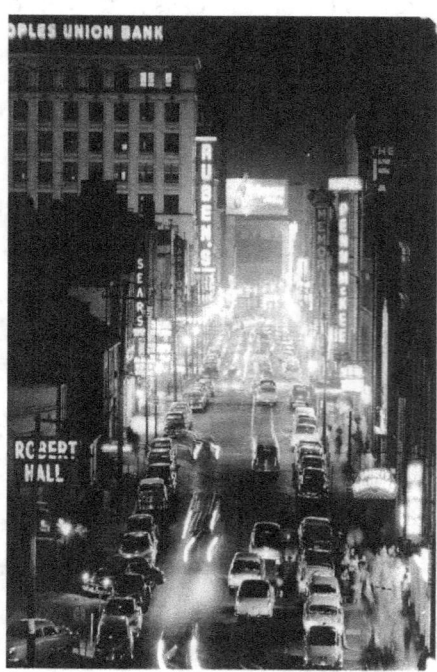

Fifth Avenue during prosperous times in the McKeesport shopping district in the Fifties.
Photo: McKeesport Regional History and Heritage Center, McKeesport, PA

In boom times, steelworkers made good money. Dad would get a pay envelope containing cash and coins from National Tube on payday. I remember that if I stole a hefty half-dollar silver coin from my father's pants pocket, I could buy 10 Reese's Peanut Butter Cups with it at the local drug store. Millions of dollars from tens of thousands of steel industry pay envelopes were spent each week in McKeesport and the rest of the Steel Valley.

Chapter 2: Marriage and a Family

In the Fifties and early Sixties, between two strikes and four recessions, downtown McKeesport could appear very prosperous. At its best, McKeesport was a symbol of the economic marvel created by the steel industry. The wide Fifth Avenue sidewalks were crowded with shoppers. The shopping district stretched for about 20 blocks along Fifth Avenue east from its terminus at the Youghiogheny River and for several blocks to the south of Fifth Avenue as well. Streetcars came by every few minutes with their bells dinging. McKeesport had heavy rail and streetcar service to Pittsburgh and streetcar service to smaller towns in the area.

As I recall, the heart of downtown had several big local department stores, a hotel, several movie theaters, two large five-and-tens, five bowling alleys, two or three pool halls, two Isaly dairy/delicatessen stores (which originated the Klondike ice cream bar), and hundreds of small shops, such as shoe, clothing, jewelry, auto accessory, and sporting goods stores. I guess that McKeesport had a population of merchants that was equal to multiple large modern shopping malls. All of these businesses drawing revenue from the steel industry in turn employed people themselves.

One of the local five-and-tens, G. C. Murphy Co., grew to a chain of 529 stores nationwide. I remember that during the Sixties, Murphy's office building in McKeesport employed hundreds of workers -- mostly young ladies -- who would stream out at lunchtime to patronize local dining establishments, including the Isaly cafeteria where I worked part-time as a teenager for 95 cents an hour.

But just as gloomy orange night skies hung over the area, so did the threats of a steel strike or "getting laid off" in a recession. Worse, there was the possibility that

Chapter 2: Marriage and a Family

unemployment compensation, simply called "unemployment," would run out during a recession, or that union support payments, called "sub pay," would be exhausted during a strike.

There were strikes in 1952 and 1959, and recessions in 1954, 1958, 1960-61, and 1969-70. I remember that my parents got angry at Republican President Dwight D. Eisenhower because he was slow to invoke the Taft Hartley Act to force striking steelworkers back to work during an especially painful strike in 1959, which lasted almost 4 months. Dad and Mary Regina were hurting financially and getting desperate. I remember going with my father one day to stand in line at the Port Vue public library in the basement of the Borough Building to pick up bags of corn meal and flour, cans of pork, and plain brown boxes of powdered milk and cheese similar to Velveeta, as the government distributed "surplus food" to families of steelworkers who were out of work.

Dad painted his father-in-law's house to get money during one such period of hard times.

When steelworkers went back to work, some faced payments on debt they had accumulated while off. There were no Visa or MasterCard accounts, but people had charge accounts at individual stores.

The 1959 strike, for example, produced a labor contract that was good only for 24 months – probably not even enough time to pay off a family's debts from the strike -- so the settlement provided little promise of future financial security. The 1959 strike was followed by a steel industry recession that some analysts believed was caused in part by steel users discovering during the strike that they

Chapter 2: Marriage and a Family

could obtain steel at lower cost from Japan and South Korea.

Steelworkers could take some comfort in knowing that they were living among people in similar circumstances. A half million steelworkers in the U.S. were idled by the 1959 strike. Steel Valley Congressman Joseph M. Gaydos had 50,000 constituents from his district working in the steel industry in 1968, according to his obituary in the *Pittsburgh Post-Gazette* newspaper. Gaydos would rant in union halls, and complain in the newspapers and on television about the dumping of cheap foreign steel into the U.S. I am pretty sure I remember Gaydos using the now politically incorrect word "Japs" in public speeches.

Problems with the steel industry, including new environmental regulations, hurt the McKeesport business district. However, downtown McKeesport also was damaged severely by the opening in 1963 of the huge Eastland suburban mall where ladies, who had just recently begun to drive cars *en masse*, did not have to search for a parking space, parallel park, or feed the parking meters, as was necessary downtown. They could park for free in a sprawling mall parking lot.

Stores closed downtown and eventually the government started urban renewal, a fiasco in which charming old structures with stone or brick facades were razed and replaced with new concrete buildings. The urban-renewal buildings also became empty relatively soon after they opened as the new occupant businesses failed too. With the devastation of the steel industry, even the Eastland mall itself closed in 2005. The population of McKeesport rose and fell from 1,392 in 1850, to a peak of 55,355 in 1940, to an estimated 19,561 in 2014.

Chapter 2: Marriage and a Family

Meanwhile, despite adversity during the changing times, Dad and Mary Regina, like the other couples of Port Vue, struggled to make a good life together. Dad – in my eyes -- represented his "Greatest Generation" well. My parents improved the asbestos home, covering the vinyl-asbestos tile floors with thick pink wall-to-wall carpeting, and upgraded their furniture. Dad finished his attic to provide a bedroom for me when my sister Jeanne was born in 1957, expanding the two-bedroom home to three. Dad did the carpentry and electrical work and installed the sheet rock, then called plaster board. He hired a plasterer and a hod carrier to finish the walls with multiple coats of plaster, including a final coat that was tinted pale yellow.

Mary Regina furnished my new room with a six- or seven-piece set of solid maple wraparound furniture, including a corner desk with a protective glass overlay and a bed with a bookcase headboard. She had good taste, but the furniture probably was expensive and it probably was put on a charge account.

Dad bought from Sears, Roebuck and Co. in downtown McKeesport a garage that had been a display sample. He dug deep trenches in the back yard and called in a concrete truck to pour level footers in the bottom of the trenches. He laid on the footers for the garage a concrete block foundation that was about 8 feet high on the low side of the sloping yard. He also dug a deep trench for a floor drain, laid in terracotta drain pipe, backfilled the trench, and poured the garage floor. Sears cut the garage into sections and delivered it. Dad, with the help of friends and relatives, reassembled the building on the foundation he had laid. It was a marvelous project.

A furious storm blew up from the airport side of the Monongahela Valley a few weeks after my father erected

Chapter 2: Marriage and a Family

the garage. During the storm, as the wind actually howled, Dad rushed out into the garage and frantically nailed two-by-four braces across the upper inside corners of the walls to keep the garage from twisting and blowing over. He was lucky to have had some spare two-by-fours on hand.

During those days Dad would have been in his late twenties or early thirties. By today's norms, he had shouldered quite a bit of responsibility and accomplished a lot by that age.

The driveway going back to the garage was made of slag, a ubiquitous glassy sand-like waste product from the steel mill blast furnaces, that the developer used to level off the lots and for driveways. Slag driveways would get ruts from the automobile tires and would harden like rock with the passage of time. Dad replaced his slag driveway with a concrete one, getting help from neighbors and relatives, including Mary Regina's brother, Jack. He also poured a patio behind the house, and then built a roof over the patio.

The couple landscaped the house nicely with shrubs and an umbrella-shaped, pink-blossoming Japanese cherry tree in the front.

Dad repeatedly drove to the nearby woods with empty bushel baskets in his car trunk, and then dug and hauled home many bushels of rich, black, top soil, which was composed mostly of decayed leaves that had accumulated undisturbed over many decades. In this soil, he raised a lush lawn. He was so serious about his lawn that he bought a Briggs & Stratton reel-type power mower instead of the usual rotary power mower with a single spinning blade that everyone else had. He believed the rotary mowers tore and damaged the blades of grass but the reel-type mowers cut them cleanly.

Chapter 2: Marriage and a Family

Mary Regina cultivated small plants and beds of flowers, including many chrysanthemums and tulips. I often saw her kneeling in the lawn digging out dandelions. The property looked nice.

Those days likely held some happiness for Dad and Mary Regina. My dad seemed to be delivering the dedication and effort expected from a husband and father, and Mary Regina instilled a sense of good taste and propriety in the household.

Thinking of those days caused me to recall the often quoted verse from the 1856 John Greenleaf Whittier poem, *Maud Muller*:

> *For of all sad words of tongue or pen,*
> *The saddest are these: "It might have been."*

I remember that my parents shared a liking for music, and Dad was a Hi Fi buff. He assembled his own H.H. Scott stereo amplifier and tuner from a kit, bought a Garrard Lab 80 turntable, and built two large speaker cabinets, full of woofers and tweeters, that he used as end tables. He had an LP album called *Paris in the Springtime* and another called *Can-Can*. On the jacket of *Paris in the Springtime* was a picture of a Parisian outdoor market with a watermelon stand and a vendor wearing a beret, which must have reminded him of his time in Paris during the war. Both Mary Regina and Dad liked the album *My Fair Lady*, and they enjoyed watching the weekly musical shows of Lawrence Welk and Mitch Miller on TV. Mary Regina liked Johnny Mathis, but Dad hated him. They had dozens of LPs.

Despite a few such pleasant memories, I could not remember truly warm and happy extended periods of good

Chapter 2: Marriage and a Family

times over the 18 years the family lived together. Maybe this was because I myself was a depressed person. Maybe I had one of those conditions that kids today are treated for, but which no one knew existed when I was a child. Or maybe I shared some genetic afflictions with my mother.

The divorce court records confirmed that Mary Regina was quite unhappy for a very long time, starting with the first year of her marriage. Mary Regina's allegations in court filings contained multiple statements in her own words (and her lawyers') to that effect: "Such conduct began immediately after the marriage . . . and continued even after the . . . filing of the (divorce) complaint." Mary Regina and her lawyers complained that after the marriage she "was continually forced to accept charity from her parents and family, for the next 17 years."

Repeated in Mary Regina's divorce complaint was the phrase "throughout the entire course of the marriage" or equivalent wording. One paragraph stated, in the words of Mary Regina and her lawyer: "The Plaintiff and Defendant engaged in quarrels and arguments continuously during the course of their marriage concerning such subjects as: his running around with other women, the raising of their son, [and] his [Dad's] refusal to seek work when he was unemployed."

Maybe there was doubt about whether Dad was guilty of some of what Mary Regina accused him of, but there was no doubt their home was not a happy one.

Dad drove a second-hand Hudson car early in the marriage. He was always having car trouble, ranging from small problems like frequent flat tires, which he fixed himself with two tire irons and innertube-patching kits, to big trouble like bad piston rings. I learned from my father

Chapter 2: Marriage and a Family

that if the smoke coming out of the exhaust pipe was black or white, that was only a sign of something minor, such as fouled spark plugs or carburetor misadjustment, but if the smoke was the dreaded color blue, that meant you needed a (piston) "ring job." The family could not afford a new car, and always had used ones.

A neighbor, Grant Ross, bought or took over management of an Atlantic gas station on U.S. Route 30 in Irwin, Pennsylvania, about 12 miles east of McKeesport. Dad, who was mechanically inclined, possessed manual dexterity, and knew all the automobile terminology, would work at the gas station for Grant pumping gas, fixing flats, mounting new tires, and doing brake jobs and tune-ups while he was on strike or laid off from the mill. Also, he would work at the gas station during days off from his steel mill job just to earn extra money.

Dad sometimes took me to the gas station with him, where I would pump gas. I was only 11 or 12 and I remember trying to conceal my youthful ineptitude when I could not find a customer's gas cap, such as on Cadillacs, which had the gas cap concealed behind a hinged tail light, or when I could not find the hood release when trying to check the oil.

According to a divorce court document, Dad worked 800 hours at the gas station one particular year. Looking back, I guessed that Dad's hours away from home at the gas station or in the mill working overtime were not good for the marriage, considering Mary Regina's suspicious nature. I wondered whether Dad took me to the gas station so that Mary Regina would have some assurance that he really was going to work.

Chapter 2: Marriage and a Family

At his main job, in the National Tube steel mill, which made drill pipe for oil wells and other types of pipe, Dad was excelling. While employed as a craneman, the high school dropout taught himself about the electrician's trade by reading books at home, or by reading during idle time at the mill. The crane cabs in the mill had ample reading material, mostly "dirty books" -- figuratively and literally (sexually explicit paperbacks or magazines that were likely to have greasy fingerprints on them) -- indicating the cranemen had considerable free time. Dad read self-improvement books.

He was an exemplary employee. When others called off work because the snow was too deep to drive through, Dad would trudge to work. Calling off was not an option for someone with his strong work ethic.

Over the years, Dad was selected to be a motor inspector in the T&P (Tube and Pipe) Electric Shop, and then as one of the relief foremen, who would fill in for the regular foremen when they were on vacation. Motor inspectors maintained electrical equipment while men called millwrights handled mechanical aspects of maintaining mill machinery.

T&P Electric Shop was responsible for getting production going again if something electrical went wrong in one of the enormous pieces of equipment on the production floor, so the job of a T&P Electric foreman was an important and challenging one. The men on the production lines operated heavy mill machinery that would pierce, lengthwise, white-hot solid steel cylinders called billets, with a series of progressively larger diameter "plugs" and "piercing bars" to make seamless pipe. Before each pass of the piercing bar through the billet, a larger diameter plug was fitted onto the end of the piercing bar,

Chapter 2: Marriage and a Family

and the pipe expanded in diameter and grew longer during each pass. Men wearing T-shirts because of the heat from the white-hot metal would throw large shovel-loads of rock salt into the pipes to lubricate the plugs between passes. When the salt entered a hot pipe, flames would flare out of the end.

On top of their hourly wages, men were paid incentive bonuses based on how many pipes they produced in a shift. When the phone rang in the T&P Electric Shop and a production foreman reported that a mill was down, workers and the company both were losing money, and the pressure was on. T&P Electric foremen were responsible for getting the mill back up and running with minimal delay.

Dad, who acquired a management point of view, told me that the thirst for incentive pay was so strong that if the production line was malfunctioning and making defective pipe, but was still able to produce pipe, the production workers sometimes would ignore the defects and continue to operate the mill. They could produce what might ultimately amount to hundreds of tons of defective pipe for the remainder of their shift just to earn their incentive pay. Later, after failing inspection, the bad pipe would be cut up, flattened in a hydraulic press, and loaded into railroad cars to be shipped to Duquesne and re-melted into billets in the Duquesne mill's furnaces. Dad called this practice "making scrap."

Danger was everywhere in the mill. The individual pipes could weigh tons, with some having walls a half inch thick (called "500 wall" for five hundred 1,000ths of an inch) and certain types of pipe could be 24 inches in diameter and 80 feet long. These pipes were often in motion, riding lengthwise on motorized roller conveyers shaped like giant steel spools, rolling on huge waist-high

Chapter 2: Marriage and a Family

table-like racks made of steel I-beams, or traveling overhead in crane "lifts" of multiple pipes hanging from steel cables or thick nylon ropes. The racks were about 3 feet above the floor and were made of I-beams spaced horizontally about 2 feet apart. Men could walk through the racks, passing between the I-beams. Pipes would rest or roll on the racks, spanning the I-beams, which were perpendicular to the pipes. Getting caught between two pipes as one rolled into another on a rack could be fatal.

The mill had a pickling pit in which acid was used to remove oxidation from the surface of steel; a soaking pit in which billets were heated (soaked with heat to 2,400 degrees) for processing; catwalks that passed near fire and smoke; and long ladders reaching up nearly to the roof that cranemen would climb to get to their overhead cranes. Workers had to shout to be heard over the noise even when standing face to face.

Along with the clanging of steel against steel, there was almost constant high-pitched noise emitted by an electric welding machine, and blaring sirens that cranemen were required to sound as they hoisted lifts of pipe and moved them overhead across the mill. Men on the floor were supposed to move out of the way when they heard a siren, because cranemen were not allowed to pass lifts directly over men. Some noise, such as that of steel striking steel when pipes were dropped into railroad cars or into storage racks, traveled for miles through the night air, sometimes all the way up into Port Vue.

This noisy environment in which so many heavy things were in motion and sometimes obscured by smoke could be disorienting.

Chapter 2: Marriage and a Family

According to an archive document posted on the internet by the University of Pittsburgh, nine men were killed among 284 who were seriously hurt in separate accidents at McKeesport's National Works during the Fifties. Reading the archived list of serious injuries that happened in that mill during the decade will make most people wince. The archive document names the victims and their injuries. Finger amputations were among the more frequent, but there were also toe and arm amputations, eye injuries, burns, and crushed ribs and a crushed skull. During the Sixties an intense safety campaign by U.S. Steel drastically reduced the death and injury rates, but working in the mill remained dangerous.

Men repairing machinery were especially vulnerable, and each such worker had his own personal padlock with his name on it, with which he was supposed to "lock out" equipment electrical panels before starting work. This precaution was intended to ensure that no one accidentally started the equipment while workmen were working on it, or in it, and that equipment did not suddenly lurch into motion on its own.

Some mill equipment ran on high amperage, 440-volt direct current (DC) that was much more likely to electrocute than the 30-amp, 110-volt alternating current (AC) used in homes. At home, Dad would work on electrical circuits while they were "hot," without bothering to remove the fuse, but he would not do that in the mill.

The nonsupervisory workers in the mill wore yellow hard hats. The relief foremen wore grey hats. The foremen wore white hats. At about the time Dad got his grey hat, he and Mary Regina began shopping for a new split-level brick home, in a new development out in the Irwin area.

Chapter 2: Marriage and a Family

"Grey hats" -- the name for the men who wore them -- were enrolled in the formal U.S. Steel management training program, and I remember Dad studying hard at home, writing answers into company instruction binders full of glossy, loose-leaf sheets printed in color. I especially remember him getting very fearful as his training classes in public speaking were approaching.

Dad eventually earned his white hat. This normally would have been a life-changing event because "white hats" were salaried management employees, not union wage employees, and they did not go on strike or get laid off. During strikes, the white hats would continue to go to work and collect their pay. If union pickets objected to foremen crossing the picket lines, the company could move temporary residence trailers into the mill and the management personnel could stay inside around the clock, performing maintenance until the atmosphere calmed down or the strike ended. Along with a white hat came financial stability and security.

Some time after being made a foreman, Dad was further selected to be schooled in the workings of the new computerized equipment, as the mills transitioned from analog to digital controls.

As a teenager I worked parts of two summers at National Tube and I observed my father's demeanor as a foreman as he interacted with the men. I think Dad said T&P Electric Shop had about 150 men. Dad was calm, quiet, and serious, but he had what the military call a "command voice" when he answered the T&P Electric Shop phone. It was clear that he was respected by his own men as well as by the production workers, though he was not necessarily liked by everyone. He had learned enough that he could competently guide subordinates about the

Chapter 2: Marriage and a Family

performance of their tasks. In any workplace there are human relations issues, but no one shared with me any negative opinions he had about my father.

One summer in the mill, I worked side by side with two black men who reminded me of the 1950s TV characters Amos 'n' Andy in skin color and size, but not in personality. One was a large man like Andy and the other a small one like Amos. I can still picture them in my mind, with their knee-length leather aprons and full-face clear-plastic shields to protect them from sparks as they ground defects out of pipe. These men treated me very well and since they were the first black people I ever interacted with, they formed the foundation for my lifelong strong respect for black working men. Though I can't remember their names, I feel some affection for these two co-workers even as I recall them in my old age.

Blacks were few in number in the National Tube steel mill in the Sixties, and I don't recall seeing any women in the mill when I worked there.

My black co-workers taught me the job of OD (outside dimension) grinder, and I did not think they treated me differently because my father was a foreman in a different department of the mill. The three of us would use industrial air grinders and abrasive disks to grind out the "scale scab" defects in finished pipe, and salvage the pipe if the grinding did not have to go too deep to remove the scale. We would taper and feather the edges of the grind area, and avoid making gouges, so the area worked on would be inconspicuous. We took some pride in our work.

We used micrometers to check the depth of the grinds, and we could be depended upon to make the right decision on whether the pipe was salvageable. Amos or Andy

Chapter 2: Marriage and a Family

marked with blue paint sticks the grinds that went too deep. Those sections of pipe would be cut out, and the remaining short pieces of good pipe would be sold. After the grinding, a crane would move the pipes to brightly lit tables made of steel girders where people employed by the buyers of the pipe would inspect them. My two black co-workers were the type of men I would love to have as co-workers or be able to hire if I had a business of my own.

(Later, because I had known "Amos" and "Andy," I did not fear mature black men when I worked in Pittsburgh's black neighborhoods as a newspaper reporter in the early 1970s. I was wary only of belligerent young toughs and drug addicts or drug dealers. I was able to distinguish between people who might be threats and those who were not. There was in fact some danger in my Pittsburgh urban work environment. My black street-wise city editor, Diane Perry, cautioned me one day to "just be patient" while we were stuck on Center Avenue, in the Hill District, waiting for the driver in front of us to finish making a drug deal from his car. "Don't blow the horn Beerman, or you will have to fight him," she warned.)

In the culture of the steel mill, some union members were militant and at odds with management. As in many workplaces, the workers sorted out along a spectrum, with some being agreeable, and others hostile. Some workers, although not all (Amos and Andy, for example, were not boisterous, coarse, or impolite), used the F word as every part of speech – noun, verb, adjective, adverb, whatever, and they could insert it into one sentence a half dozen times. Using such language was habit forming. Because of the noise in the mill, workers often had to shout these obscenities as they communicated.

Chapter 2: Marriage and a Family

A few workers seemed content to do little for the company, unless incentive pay was involved. They were uncaring about the costs of steel production and the necessity for competitive pricing, and they seemed to feel no guilt about being unproductive.

For a time, because of my small size, I had a job as an ID (inside dimension) grinder. I would lie belly-down on a wheeled mechanic's creeper that was curved to fit the inside of a 24-inch-diameter pipe, and pull myself into the pipe. The pipe could be as long as 80 feet. The pipes I worked on for this job were made from long strips of steel that were unrolled from a coil and bent into a tubular shape. The length-wise seam of the resulting tube was welded by an automatic welding machine. My job was to grind smooth with an air grinder any defective lumpy weld-bead formed when a malfunctioning welding machine melted too much metal.

I had to wear fireproof clothing, headgear, gloves, goggles, and a respirator, because while the grinder was running, sparks would swirl around the inside of the pipe, making an orange ring that looked like fire when viewed by someone looking into the end of the pipe. This job was done on night shift, 11 p.m. to 7 a.m.

ID grinders worked in pairs. The concept was that one man was stationed outside the pipe, ready to turn off a valve in the air hose in case the man inside the pipe caught on fire while operating the air grinder. In practice though, sometimes the job of the man inside the pipe was to sleep and the job of the worker outside the pipe was to turn <u>on</u> the air, and consequently start the grinder, if a boss came around on night shift. The startup of the grinder would wake up the team member sleeping inside the pipe and alert

Chapter 2: Marriage and a Family

him that a boss was around. Bosses rarely came around on night turn.

Similarly, workers were cautious about switching on the lights in the locker room at night, because the room might be full of men sleeping on the benches.

A pair of full-time crane inspectors inspected three cranes a day -- two in the morning and one in the afternoon. Based on my limited observations, an inspection seemed to take less than 1 hour. Crane operators would get annoyed because inspectors would kill time sitting on the bench in the crane cab that was intended for use by the operator.

During the daylight shift, idle workers were advised to hide somewhere, and not loaf out in the open. One of my schoolmates, a fellow low-value "college kid" temporary summer employee, sometimes would come to work, clock in, and go outside to tan himself on the riverbank. This young man, who was named Dennis, had a sticker depicting the "Dennis the Menace" cartoon character on the front of his yellow hard hat.

Nevertheless, I respected steelworkers. After all, they did produce the products that the company sold, and from National Works, they supplied the oil fields with pipe. The mere idea of making a seamless pipe from a solid cylinder of steel, which itself was made from iron ore dug from the earth, and other ingredients, was amazing. Even more amazing was that the product would conform with strict engineering tolerances and technical specifications. Practically speaking, for example, some types of pipe had threaded ends, and when workmen in the field tried to thread one pipe into another on an oil drilling rig, the threads had better mate smoothly.

Chapter 2: Marriage and a Family

Of course, steelworkers also supplied other industries, including construction and auto-making, with beams and coils of sheet steel, and thousands of other products. Highly visible proof that the industry made staggering amounts of money was the 64-story landmark U.S. Steel Building skyscraper, once the grandest building in Pittsburgh. Now the building bears the name of UPMC, for the University of Pittsburgh Medical Center.

Most of the National Works jobs were challenging and required skill. For example, I was assigned to operate an end facer machine. It had a control panel with green, red, white, and black buttons, and lights and dials. I was supposed to use this control panel to bring in a pipe from the holding table, and route it via conveyer rollers to the end facer machine. Then I was supposed to make the machine grip the pipe, and start a spinning ring of cutting tools that would finish the end of the pipe, leaving the end with a shiny beveled face where welders in the field would weld one pipe to the next.

As the machine made its cut, it would spin off coiled cuttings that resembled razor wire or concertina wire. As operator, I was required to change the cutting tools when they got dull, and I periodically also had to call a crane to lift away the cuttings. I was unable to become productive in this job in a reasonable time, so I was replaced diplomatically with an experienced, competent worker.

Foremen were in conflict situations. They had to get their jobs done in a culture in which some union workers harbored hostility toward the company. Foremen had to issue a quota of "white slip" citations each month, and impose a certain number of days off without pay as penalties for safety violations or other improper conduct,

Chapter 2: Marriage and a Family

such as being late, while maintaining working relationships with their subordinates.

Dad seemed to have a disposition well suited to this job. He was relaxed and confident in his competence. He was not abusive, but he was not chummy either, except with his fellow foremen. He didn't like having to fill his quota of white slips.

After becoming a foreman, Dad joined a management club bowling team, called the "Polish Republicans," a deliberate oxymoron, and he began to play golf occasionally at the Youghiogheny Country Club. As the son of a steelworker, I saw playing golf as a status symbol. Ward Cleaver, the perfect upper middle class father in the *Leave It to Beaver* TV series, played golf. Dad's career prospects seemed bright to me, considering that he was beginning to play golf, like Ward Cleaver.

When later I would hear journalist Tom Brokaw's term, "The Greatest Generation," I would think of World War II, and my father, who was just a soldier -- not a war hero. I would think also about how my father overcame obstacles such as depression-era poverty, the lack of a high school education, and his bad marriage and divorce ordeal to become a productive member of society who helped build America. Conceivably, if not for limitations associated with Dad's background and circumstances, he might have moved up the next rung of the ladder to become general foreman, I thought.

***

Unfortunately, during Dad's "gray hat" days, by the time my parents' financial situation was about to stabilize, their marriage ended. In Dad's account of the final breakup,

Chapter 2: Marriage and a Family

facing mounting bills, Mary Regina bailed out as a layoff was approaching. This happened right before Dad got his white hat, which my mother and father had not known for sure that he would get.

The jealousy problem aside, Dad said Mary Regina told him as a recession loomed that she could not go through another layoff. So, she left, and much of the money he made as a foreman went to Mary Regina's multiple divorce lawyers over 13 years, and to court costs, Internal Revenue Service audits that Mary Regina instigated, and to the cost of attempting unsuccessfully to fund two households. In those days, many women did not work, and the male routinely was responsible for all divorce costs, even for paying the opposing divorce lawyers.

I later wondered whether Mary Regina became so irrationally hostile toward Dad because she felt superior to him and wrongly believed she had married beneath herself. Maybe she was enraged by the suspicion that a high school dropout whom she considered to be inferior had the gall to cheat on her. I also thought that possibly her leaving was an attempt to bluff and gain some reassurance that he loved her, if he would ask her to come back. But he stopped asking.

***

My home life shaped me as much as the genes I inherited from my parents, and influenced my life well into adulthood. Along with what I learned about my parents' ugly divorce proceedings, long-term psychological and emotional damage I sustained in other ways during my youth formed virtual scar tissue and callouses, and kept me from ever bonding closely with my mother.

Chapter 2: Marriage and a Family

As I thought back over my childhood 6 decades later, I primarily recalled being confined as a little boy to a gloomy house alone with a very unhappy woman.

The most prominent memories of my childhood were recollections of my mother spending substantial parts of days, weeks, months, and years sitting sideways on a chair at the dining room table with her back against the wall, her knees tucked up, and her heels on the seat of the chair. She had a burning cigarette in her right hand and a coffee cup and a glass ash tray containing Pall Mall butts on the table to her left. She stared into space or across the room at the living room picture window between puffs and sips as smoke wafted around her. She gnawed her fingernails down to the quick. Dad would be at work.

I did not know the reason for Mary Regina's despondency. As I grew older I wondered whether it was some sort of a paranoia or anxiety disorder and of course, depression: paranoia regarding suspicions over what Dad was doing when he wasn't home, especially when he was supposed to be working overtime; and depression about her perceived state of her marriage, her economic situation and surroundings, her health, and her "looks." She felt she had become too "skinny" and would have the milkman deliver pint bottles of heavy cream that she hoped would help her put on some weight.

A bipolar disorder, or manic depression, was another condition that, as a layman, I later suspected my mother had suffered from. When a neighbor would show up at the door for a visit, Mary Regina went through a snap personality change. She would go from miserable to affable, as if a switch had been flipped.

Chapter 2: Marriage and a Family

Eventually I would ascribe my mother's conditions primarily to Addison's disease and thyroid cancer that were not diagnosed early enough or treated effectively. She could have had other afflictions that medical science, or her individual doctors, were not aware of at the time.

I resolved that in my own marriages, I would not act as my mother had in hers. When my first wife and I got divorced after 17 years, we reached our own settlement, without lawyers or recriminations, through New Jersey's do-it-yourself process, rather than fight it out tooth and nail in the courts as Mary Regina had done.

I recognized that I had an inclination to think like Mary Regina, especially in my second marriage, which is still ongoing after 26 years. In my first marriage, which ended suddenly, I had had no serious suspicions about spousal infidelity, but they would have been justified if I had. My first wife really was unfaithful. So in my second marriage, I had to worry about whether things I occasionally suspected really were happening, as, I discovered, they had been in my first marriage. On the other hand, sometimes I thought that maybe I was just imagining things, as I believed my mother had done.

I eventually developed some feeling for how painful jealous suspicion can be, and some empathy for what my mother had suffered.

***

Regarding interaction between my parents, I remember primarily the atmosphere. My mother would answer my father's questions or comments with the silent treatment, or with the single-syllable utterance, "Humph." There was no calm discussion of their problems, at least not that I knew

Chapter 2: Marriage and a Family

of. I wondered whether my mother's refusal to talk was because she knew she lacked factual support for her accusations or suspicions and therefore could not articulate a rational verbal complaint or argument.

Among a few bits of conversation from my parents that I remember was my father complaining that because Mary Regina did not get up until 11 a.m., the family did not go out and make good use of his days off, such as by taking a drive to Deep Creek, Maryland, or to Shawnee State Park in Pennsylvania, which he liked to do.

I also remember that once, immediately upon Dad's arrival at home after work, Mary Regina told him, "You'd better do something with that kid upstairs (me)." Dad protested, "What do you want me to do, go up and smack him around? I'm not even mad at him."

***

I could not imagine what I could have done at age 9 or 10 or younger to make my mother so dissatisfied with me. She would tell me repeatedly, and not in a joking way, "I hope your kids are just like you." Maybe she was comparing me to her brothers, who seemed like they probably had been well-behaved children.

Mary Regina would frequently threaten me, "I'm going to get the ironing cord." The "ironing" cord actually was a braided cloth-insulated electrical cord that was detachable from a waffle iron. She would use it to coerce, or, occasionally, to whip me. One day when I was a preschooler she was chasing me with the ironing cord when I dove into an upholstered chair, and hit my head on the wooden frame under the upholstery. I cut my scalp, and the gash bled profusely, staining the upholstery with blood.

Chapter 2: Marriage and a Family

Mary Regina had to have a neighbor drive her and me to McKeesport Hospital, as she held me on her lap and pressed a compress on my head. At the hospital my head was stitched up. When Dad got home from work, he saw that I had a big white bandage on my head. I cannot remember Dad's reaction but it certainly would have been minimal. After all, the stitches were more the result of an accident than abuse.

Nevertheless, today Mary Regina might be reported to a child welfare agency by someone on the McKeesport Hospital staff.

Almost everyone believed in corporal punishment in the Fifties and Sixties, including teachers, especially nuns and priests teaching in Catholic schools. I grew up believing in it too. It kept the kids behaving appropriately, most importantly in the schools, and the classroom discipline allowed them to get a good education. However, later I was very limited in what I could do regarding parental discipline, since my kids were taught in school to say, "I'm gonna call DYFS (pronounced die-fiss)," which stood for Division of Youth and Family Services in New Jersey, where they grew up.

The real pain in my childhood did not come from corporal punishment. It came from loneliness and the unhappy home environment. I spent my earliest years living out each day with my downhearted mother, who had little to say to me, except for giving warnings or orders, like, "Wait till your father gets home," "Eat your breakfast," or "Go get your bath."

Early on, a boy who was my age lived next door, and we would play in our back yards in the summer, catching grasshoppers and bees in glass jars with air holes punched

Chapter 2: Marriage and a Family

in the lids, digging with metal toy construction equipment, or building tiny bridges for toy trucks in the dirt with mud and Popsicle sticks. These were a few good days when I had someone to talk to. But my friend's family moved to the next town after a short time.

Later, as a parent myself, I felt that companionship was very important for young children. I knocked on doors in my new neighborhood of Mount Ephraim, N.J., to introduce myself to neighbors and arrange for playmates for my daughter, Heidi, who then was age 4.

I myself spent thousands of hours as a child lying on the floor watching snowy, low resolution, black-and-white TV on a set connected to rabbit ears or later to a roof antenna. It actually was difficult to even make out what was happening on the screen. Occasionally the vertical hold control would fail, and the picture would repeatedly roll up and off the screen from the bottom. Sometimes I could stop the rolling by adjusting a dial on the front of the set.

There were only three commercial TV channels and the educational station, which was on the air only part of each day. I watched *Howdy Doody*, *The Lone Ranger*, *Roy Rogers*, *Zorro*, the *Cisco Kid*, and *Superman*. Most of these shows used the same scenery in every episode and I could tell many of the scenes were filmed in the studio with fake backgrounds.

I was alone with my mother in a world of irrelevant, mostly boring, TV fiction. I could have benefitted from some of today's advanced, upbeat, children's TV shows. There was no *Sesame Street* back then.

I spent 9 years as what was commonly called "an only child," and even after my sister was born, the age gap was

Chapter 2: Marriage and a Family

too great for us to be companions. It would not have been so bad being an only child if the adult in the household had engaged with me in conversation.

Later I would think of the case of Jacob, the orphan cat from Alberta, Canada, in the internet video, who was raised by Esperanza, the Husky dog, as part of a litter of puppies. Jacob the cat grew up thinking he was a dog, and acting like one. Raised alone, I had no role model except my depressed mother and I didn't have a clue about how a kid should act.

I think this near-solitary-confinement environment over a period of many years left me naïve and always behind the other kids in social development.

I never fully recovered and sometimes in my old age looking back I am amazed that I was able to earn my way through life, without ever getting fired, and qualify for a pension. I felt that I must have done it by working much harder than other people to compensate for my poor perception of reality and utter incompetence at office politics.

As an adult office worker lacking good situational awareness, I was astounded that I repeatedly came to be one of the last to know about various extramarital affairs that went on in the workplace among my coworkers. I also was slow to be convinced when coworkers gossiped that certain employees were gay. This further undermined my confidence in my perception of the world around me. Although learning of the affairs generally affected my degree of respect for the participants, discovering that someone was gay did not. I never knew a gay individual that I had reason to dislike. Actually, I disliked those who gossiped and joked about gay people.

Chapter 2: Marriage and a Family

* * *

I turned 6 years old on October 1, but Mary Regina persuaded the nuns to enroll me in first grade even though the cutoff was age 6 by September 1. I had not been to kindergarten, which put me at a disadvantage to any of the children who had been there. As a result of my early start in first grade, some of my classmates were older chronologically by 13 months. One classmate who lived a block from me was 25 months older than I because he had been held back ("flunked") a grade. As we grew older, the two of us would walk home from school together and we hung out as friends in seventh, eighth, and ninth grades. This socially advanced older friend eventually introduced me to some loose girls in the nearby town of Glassport, but I didn't know what to do with them and I also was constrained by religious concerns.

As an adult I wondered whether Mary Regina had been eager to get me into first grade just to get me out of the house. Many parents today hope to send their kids off to kindergarten, prekindergarten, or nursery school, so the parents can go to work, or for other reasons. To look at it another way, though, I wondered whether preschool and kindergarten might have helped me by getting me out of a depressing home earlier, and would have put me closer to par with the other kids, assuming we were all the same age.

Mary Regina would brag occasionally that a nun suggested I was intelligent enough to skip a grade in my early years in elementary school, but I eventually realized I was very lucky that this had not happened. I believed I should have been held back a grade instead, not only because I was usually the smallest kid -- boy or girl -- in my class, but because I just did not feel I was in harmony socially with the other kids.

Chapter 2: Marriage and a Family

I did not understand what was going on around me. Lack of situational awareness seems to be the best way to describe it, using today's terminology. Because of my isolated home life, I was not used to hearing kids around me engage in conversation. If a wisecrack or joke was directed at me, I just didn't get it. I was slow to grasp or I missed completely verbal or visual cues that my classmates could pick up.

Being shorter than almost all of the girls in my class in seventh and eighth grades drastically limited my pool of potential girlfriends. The fact that I really "liked" a few of the girls made this situation painful.

Finally, when I got to be 10 or 11, I became friends with some of my male classmates and I was allowed to walk or ride my bicycle to their homes five or six blocks away.

We would sneak off to explore an abandoned coal mine tunnel; look for pop bottles at the town dump, for which we could collect 2 cents in deposit refunds for 6-ounce bottles or a nickel for quart bottles; walk to the penny candy store; flip baseball cards; swing on a cable hanging from a tree over a ravine in the woods; take long bike rides; and play pickup baseball and football. Those days were just like those depicted in the movie, *Stand by Me*, which is set in 1959, when I would have been 11. The movie is based on the Stephen King novella, *The Body*. My friends and I actually found a dead body. It was a shaggy, rotting, maggoty carcass of a big mongrel dog who was lying on his side at the garbage dump. We poked at him with sticks.

I held mild grudges about decisions that Mary Regina made about me, such as entering me early into first grade,

Chapter 2: Marriage and a Family

which I felt significantly affected my development. Mary Regina would not allow me to play organized football because, she said, I was too small. However, I could run faster than probably every kid my age in the town and I was adept at juking tacklers. I thought that if my mother had not prevented me, I could have been a good halfback. I knew of other halfbacks on organized teams who were small like me. I did well in and enjoyed tackle football pickup games. I was tough enough. I would have enjoyed the comradery of being part of an organized football team, and that could have had a big influence on my developing personality.

As for baseball, my solitary early childhood gave me no baseball skill, and, at entry level age, I could not make the town baseball teams. I remember that when a few kids were left unpicked after team selections by the coaches, the town's men decided to create another team for the left-behinds, then called "wastes" by the other kids. To my humiliation, I was not even picked for the leftovers team. Mary Regina reinforced my embarrassment by expressing in front of a neighbor her amazement that I was rejected for the scrubs team. She was focusing on the neighbor, rather than on me. She never talked directly to me one-on-one about such things.

Later, I developed solid baseball skills in non-league play after the town bulldozed a dirt field into a strip-mined area near my home and I spent many days playing there. I had just been a year or two behind everyone else, and lacking in experience, but I caught up.

(My youth sports memories influenced my behavior as a parent. As a father in Haddon Heights, N.J., I installed a pitcher's mound and a home plate in my back yard, and coached my son one on one. The coaching brought out a talent for pitching. Bill Junior could throw about 28 strikes

Chapter 2: Marriage and a Family

out of 30 hard and fast pitches in a typical practice session at age 10. The other pitchers at that age couldn't get the ball over the plate, but Bill Junior could force batters to either hit or strike out, rather than draw a walk. He impressed the coaches at the end of his season as a 10-year-old, and one coach told him he had been "noticed." But the next season the coaches forgot about him and used their own kids as pitchers. My son instead played third base. He stuck with baseball long enough to find out he was capable of hitting soaring home runs.

(I also supported my son as he played 10 years of travel-team ice hockey. I took him to practices two or three times a week, and to games all over New Jersey and southeastern and central Pennsylvania on Saturdays and Sundays. Similarly, I attended my daughter's cheerleading competitions and softball games.)

One summer at about age 12, I went swimming almost every day at the Glassport public swimming pool. I was hanging out then with two Polish classmates who were twins and a year older. The boys were becoming interested in girls, and girls found the blondish twins attractive. The twins and I would rub on baby oil with iodine mixed in it to improve our tans, and lift weights in the twins' basement to build our muscles. The twins had as a role model in their strength-building exercises an older brother. Besides lifting weights, he would hammer copper nails part-way into the basement ceiling joists and then bend them over with his bare fingers.

One day the twins decided to further lighten their hair by combing peroxide through it. I of course participated in this. The twins were part of a normal family, and if they thought something was okay, I didn't give it a second thought. Actually, the question of right or wrong did not enter my mind regarding the peroxide. The results did not show up immediately and I put on too much. My brown hair turned orange blond. Today orange blond hair on a male would be an indicator of possible gayness or punkiness. In those days it simply meant queer. But I was either too young or too naïve to know what queer was. Mary Regina surely knew and she undoubtedly was concerned.

Unfortunately, there was no discussion of such things in the Beerman home; mostly just silence.

I suffered some abuse from older boys because of my hair, although I was unaware as to what their real issue was. Suburban America was more macho and violent then. Verbal and physical assaults were common. Some coaches would curse at young team members and even manhandle them, and young boys and even girls would fight at the slightest provocation. So, I didn't think it especially strange that some kids harassed me.

Many of the boys were sons of tattooed war veterans who were aggressively assertive of their masculinity. Boys played war, wearing their fathers' helmets, canteens, mess kits, tactical belts, folding foxhole shovels called entrenching tools, and other military equipment brought back from the war. They would do belly crawls under imaginary barbed wire, and throw imaginary grenades. They played at hand-to-hand combat, as well as with imaginary bayonets, rifles, and handguns. Some kids had learned judo maneuvers such as takedowns from their fathers. As the boys grew older, exuding testosterone, real fistfights became common.

The peroxide event was one of many instances in which I naively became a victim of circumstances. I later

Chapter 2: Marriage and a Family

wondered why my mother or father had not simply advised me to shave my head or at least get a crew cut to get rid of the orange hair. In normal families, brothers and sisters would have instantly attacked me on the subject of my hair at the dinner table during the very first meal. Instead, my mother's suppressed or silent way of reacting turned what could have been an episode in a situation comedy like *Leave It to Beaver* into an extended stressful experience with a stigma that endured even after the roots grew out.

I realized later as an adult that my father had not been home much and had not provided help or advice to me during my elementary and high school years, although he would be a good friend later.

I would be isolated again -- this time outside the home -- when Mary Regina insisted I enroll in the new regional Catholic all-boys high school, Serra High School. Beginning at age 12, I was bused every morning along with a handful of other kids out of Port Vue to a school about 6 miles away in the Haler Heights section of McKeesport. This separated me from my grade school classmates, such as the twins, almost all of whom went to the public high school. It also kept me from developing the social comfort, graces, and skills that I presumed would come from going to a co-ed high school, which I considered to be normal high school.

Many Port Vue boys became overtly hostile toward Serra High School students, including me, because the Serra friars lured away some of the leading basketball and football athletes from the local public schools by waiving their tuition.

I blamed my mother for sending me to Serra, a school like the one she had attended, although later I could see that

Chapter 2: Marriage and a Family

I had gained some benefits from going to a Catholic high school.

Eventually I formed some high school friendships. In particular, I welcomed and made friends with a student who had relocated over the summer to McKeesport from California. We ended up hanging out at the pool hall together, and double dating with our respective girlfriends, for about 3 years until he joined the Navy and got married.

I also fell into an extended relationship with a nice girl, herein called Bill's Girlfriend (BG), who became a light in my life during the dark days of my youth.

I dated BG for years, and we went steady on and off. She had a very nice family, including an older sister and brother, and she and her family treated me very well. BG and her mother would feed me, frequently cooking hamburgers and French fries. BG, her parents, and I would all sit together and watch TV shows such as the Carol Burnett Show when BG and I came home early from dates. BG's older brother took me on a trip with him to the Can-Am Mid-Ohio sports car race.

BG, a trim, shapely, somewhat petite, green-eyed blonde, looked fine enough to give a boy a lump in his throat; she could not have been any more attractive. She also was smart, had a pleasant personality, and constantly displayed a smile. She was a standout even at a large regional high school where the majority of the girls were attractive.

BG and I would do the usual things like go to the soda fountain, or double date for miniature golf. She tried unsuccessfully to teach me to dance in preparation for a high school semiformal. Once or twice we went to church together, at her suggestion.

We spent dozens of evenings together at the Greater Pittsburgh or Rainbow Gardens drive-in theaters, or parking at "The Ranch" lover's lane under the McKeesport-Duquesne Bridge, listening to Motown on the car radio. Sometimes we would take her dad's car, which had fold-down seats. I would never forget the intoxicating fragrance of her Heaven Scent perfume, and she was heaven-sent to me. She was a dream girl, although I did not fully realize it then.

Although she was playful, she would not give in to me, saying she wanted to be a virgin when she got married. Most girls were "good girls" in the Sixties, at least that's what I thought.

When my classmates at Penn State first used the expression "blue balls," the words were new to me, but I understood instantly what they meant. I knew how painful a prolonged state of arousal could become.

Looking back, I think I was too immature for BG, even though she was 2 years younger, and that my conduct was sometimes asinine and intolerable. I simply did not have my head together. When she finally broke up with me, it ripped out my heart. The breakup taught me that pain does not come only from physical injuries.

BG always was getting hit on. Pursuers included a golden boy halfback and a burly brute of a tackle from the high school football team, and a sailor who would visit her when he was on leave. Once, she got pulled over by a traffic cop who wanted her phone number. Looking at old

Chapter 2: Marriage and a Family

photos, anyone could see that she was beautiful, and that I was not in her league. I wondered what she ever saw in me.

Maybe she thought I had potential, and broke off the relationship with finality after I graduated from college with a degree in journalism, and she concluded that in fact I did not have potential. Ironically, I thought my college graduation photos of us together, with me in my suit, at Beaver Stadium in State College were the only ones in which I looked okay. My poor ability for accurate situational awareness prevented me from fully understanding the beginning, middle, and end of the relationship.

BG eventually bought herself a yellow Corvette, if I recall correctly, and I thought of her when I saw Christie Brinkley in the blonde-in-a-sports-car scene in the movie, *National Lampoon Vacation*.

For the most part, my time with her was very good, and if not for this mostly positive part of my youth, my life back then would have been devoid of happiness and self-esteem. I would have missed a lot. I guess now that very few of my high school classmates had been lucky enough to have had a girlfriend experience as good as mine.

Many years later, I was blessed to meet and marry a girl who was much like BG, although that is not what attracted me to her. We met at a Parents Without Partners meeting.

Martha Elba Del Avellano is not a blonde like BG, but rather a 115-pound flawlessly bilingual Latina brunette. When she was younger, she looked like Marlo Thomas, *That Girl*, in the TV series, or sometimes, to me, like

Chapter 2: Marriage and a Family

actress Natalie Wood in her role as Maria in *West Side Story*.

Martha talks to me constantly and smiles all the time, like BG. Martha even smiles while talking on the phone. It doesn't matter that the person on the other end cannot see her. That amazes me.

Martha is so smart that she makes me feel mentally deficient (to use politically correct words) in comparison. As she astounds me with her intellectual abilities, I feel dull and wonder if I am acquiring Alzheimer's disease. But then I remember that I have always been like this, and don't seem to be getting any worse, so I am reassured. Everybody likes Martha. She is my opposite, and she creates a home environment that is the antithesis of the one I grew up in. At age 68, living with Martha, a dog, and four cats, I have never been happier.

***

I can remember my mother getting upset when my father would break the news about an impending steel strike or layoff. Instead of being supportive, she would express disgust. In turn, Dad would complain, asking why Mary Regina had to shop in downtown Pittsburgh at the department stores, where she would go with her mother. He would ask, couldn't she buy inexpensive things, particularly clothes, instead of running up the charge account balance at Kaufmann's department store?

I had some sympathy for my father's complaints, because while the other kids went to St. Joseph Elementary School in inexpensive chino pants, I was sent in expensive wool dress pants. At elementary school age I did not care what I was wearing. I would rip the knees out of my pants

Chapter 2: Marriage and a Family

once or twice a week in falls during recess, and I had to go home and face my mother, who would get very upset. Mary Regina would have Grandma patch the pants on her sewing machine during our regular Sunday visits.

In contrast, when I went to high school at the regional Catholic school, clothes mattered. Many classmates had money to buy Gant shirts, wool flannel and herringbone sports coats, and Canoe cologne at the upscale men's store, Henry B. Klein's, who called themselves "Clothiers and Haberdashers." The clothes were like Brooks Brothers' clothes. I could buy some of the peer-approved clothing on installments at Klein's, but really couldn't dress up to the level of the well-to-do kids. Some of the students were the sons of doctors, lawyers, engineers, architects, and businessmen. Of course, some of the boys were mean, and some Klein's patrons would ridicule students suspected of shopping at Kadar's clothing store, another store in downtown McKeesport, which lacked their approval.

***

None of the Serra High School faculty took any interest in me. To be fair, I couldn't say the faculty took special interest in rich kids either. I just walked from class to class and sat at the desks for 4 years, not grasping what high school was all about. I would read Ian Fleming's *James Bond* paperbacks in class. I identified not with the good students, but with kids who smoked in the janitor's room, and occasionally played hooky. I was one of the kids who copied other kids' homework. When I tried to study at home at nights, it just wouldn't sink in, and I would fall asleep.

Chapter 2: Marriage and a Family

After a friend and I stole the final exam in trigonometry from the faculty room, we had to ask a smart kid to work out the problems for us.

I finished high school with an overall C average but somehow managed to get accepted into Duquesne University, a Catholic school, and to Penn State. The admissions officials must have believed a C from Serra Catholic High School was better than a C from a public school.

I also finished Penn State with a C average. I remained troubled while at Penn State, but later, in my many post-graduate courses, including my work on my master's degree from Drexel, I compiled a nearly perfect 3.9 grade point average. I also succeeded in passing the 2-day Institute of Internal Auditors' Certified Internal Auditor exam, which had a very low pass rate at the time.

Maybe I had in common with my mother that we both did better after the family home broke up and we put our past lives behind us.

***

At every age level, things I did wrong were calamities at home.

Once when I received a bad report card in high school, I was so afraid to take it home that I withheld it from my parents. In desperation, I typed up my own replacement report card and mailed it home. I ran the envelope through a postage meter owned by a businessman parent of a classmate to make the letter look authentic. I included a note saying the school's computer was broken down so the report cards for the marking period had been prepared manually. I didn't know whether I had gotten away with

Chapter 2: Marriage and a Family

this, but my parents never said anything, so I assumed I probably had.

As noted earlier, Mary Regina cited differences in how she and my dad felt about disciplining me as part of her complaint for divorce. Mary Regina would tell me, "You need to have your head examined." I never took her as being serious, but maybe she was. I learned later as an adult that Mary Regina did in fact take her aging mother to have her head examined.

Near the end of my parents' marriage, as I was about to graduate from high school, the friar who taught physics announced that he would flunk a dozen or so seniors who had not done satisfactory term projects. One physics project turned in by two football players partnering up on the project consisted of a Quaker Oats cylindrical cereal carton with a balloon in it, which the students presented as a model of a human lung. This term project would have been bad enough if one student had turned it in, but because two claimed credit for it as a joint project, the friar must have found it doubly offensive.

The physics teacher was a tall, thin, stern-looking gray-haired friar who wore rimless glasses and dressed in the brown robe of St. Francis. He probably was one of the more respected and feared teachers at the school. He reportedly was sufficiently annoyed by his students' failure to exercise due diligence on their projects that he did in fact flunk a dozen or so seniors. Failing physics prevented the students from graduating and they had to attend summer school. I thought I was likely to flunk physics too, but somehow, I escaped this fate, and got a 70, the minimum passing grade, for the semester.

Chapter 2: Marriage and a Family

After the graduation ceremony, at which some students reportedly were given certificates of attendance rather than diplomas, grandfather John Fisher snatched my diploma folder from my hand and looked inside. Apparently Mary Regina had tipped off John that there might not be a diploma in the folder, and John must have been surprised to see a diploma. I later speculated that the school had warned the parents of failing students with a phone call and in response my father had driven to the school and persuaded the physics teacher to pass me. I wondered if he had told the teacher that if I didn't graduate, there was a potential for a very serious domestic disturbance at the Beerman home.

***

Though Mary Regina's disposition normally was passive depression, there were flare-ups. The most intense fight at home that I remember was a shouting episode at night after I had gone to bed. During the argument, there was a booming crash in the kitchen that seemed to shake one end of the house. The next morning I saw a 12-inch cast iron skillet on the floor, below where it had hit a wall. The handle was broken off and was lying next to the skillet. Later I learned from my father that my mother had thrown the skillet at him. In another incident, which was cited in the initial divorce complaint, Dad slapped Mary Regina after she threw a cup of coffee at him. To my knowledge, this is the only time he touched her.

I remember my mother would tell my father, "Get away," as they were sitting on the couch together, or "Get out," meaning "Get away." As I grew older and went through one marriage and into another, I could understand how Dad must have felt while continually being spurned.

Chapter 2: Marriage and a Family

***

One of the greatest ironies that I witnessed during my life was what happened to the relationship between my sister, who was 9 years younger than I, and my father. Mary Regina displayed no affection toward either of her children at home. I thought this was manifested in the way my mother fixed my sister's hair. Mary Regina did not do it gently and lovingly, but pulled and brushed it roughly, causing pain. But Dad treasured his daughter. She was Daddy's little girl. Father and daughter would share the recliner chair in the living room, with Dad holding Jeanne in his lap as they watched TV.

After Mary Regina left, taking Jeanne with her, I called my father one day to ask for a ride, after I had hitchhiked most of the way home from Penn State. When my father picked me up, he was crying. He passed a letter to me, and blurted, "I've lost Jeanne."

In the letter, Jeanne told her father she hated him and called him a pig. This was one of the more stressful occurrences in my life. It was rivaled by another one on Christmas day, 1968, when Dad and I went to my grandparents' house on Tolma Avenue in Dormont where Mary Regina and Jeanne were living after Mary Regina had left Dad. Dad and I wanted to give Christmas presents to Jeanne, and I had one for my mother, but Mary Regina turned the visit into an extremely disturbing emotional scene.

I remember Mary Regina following Dad around, holding a tape recorder microphone in his face, as he tried to talk with his daughter during the holiday visit. I don't remember what anyone was saying during this nightmare-

Chapter 2: Marriage and a Family

like event. Perhaps my mind has blocked out details of the terrible memory.

On another occasion, Dad parked at the top of Tolma Avenue to try to see Jeanne as she walked home from school. Mary Regina or her father John called the Dormont police on Dad.

Such incidents, especially the Christmas one, led me to shy away from visits with my mother and sister for years. My godmother, Jean, my cousin, Freddie, my former girlfriend, BG, and my father attended my college graduation. I didn't invite my mother.

I invited neither my father nor my mother to my wedding because I dreaded dealing with the drama involving my parents. Actually, I even chose to avoid a normal wedding altogether because of my difficult family situation. I asked Father Donald McIlvane, a civil rights activist priest I met while working in Pittsburgh's Hill District as a newspaper reporter, to marry my fiancé and me quietly. But Father McIlvane, though willing to perform the marriage, urged me to instead get married at my fiancée's parish, Sacred Heart Church in Shadyside.

My fiancée and I did opt for a ceremony in the Sacred Heart chapel and a very small reception at her home. In retrospect, it eventually became obvious to me that I should have invited both of my parents to the wedding and let them manage their own interpersonal issues.

Such were some of the ramifications of what I considered to be my mother's mental health problems and distorted view of reality. Of course, these examples were minor compared to the cumulative long-term effects on young Jeanne's teenage years, the family's finances, and

Chapter 2: Marriage and a Family

the futures of each family member. Because I was estranged from my sister after my mother left, I knew little about her thoughts and experiences. But I did know that my sister had been prevented from knowing her father, and her relatives on her father's side of the family.

As an adult, I stayed with Jeanne at Mary Regina's apartment one night while Mary Regina was hospitalized, and I told my sister then about our father's feelings about her. I did not speak in a negative way about our mother. Jeanne had little to say. Later, while Mary Regina was dying in a nursing home, I spent some time with my brother-in-law, then a widower, who expressed surprise at my version of my parents' breakup. "You mean <u>she</u> left <u>him</u>?" he asked incredulously.

As described earlier, Dad was very successful at overcoming the handicaps and limitations in his background. So, if not for Mary Regina's decision to leave and begin a long obsession with divorce courts that was financially ruinous to the family as well as severely damaging in many intangible ways, the family would have had a comfortable financial situation and each member might have had a better life in some respects. This made me think that couples should be very cautious about making decisions to go to war against each other.

On the other hand, Mary Regina seemed to be happier in her post-marriage life. I wondered whether this was (1) because of improvement in her medical condition as she was treated with hydrocortisone for the Addison's disease and Synthroid for the Thyroid disease, (2) because she had been reborn in the quiet Catholic fashion, or (3) simply because Dad, whom she hated, was out of her life.

Chapter 3: Divorce

Mary Regina left the family home in Port Vue on Saturday, July 27, 1968, with her daughter, Jeanne, age 11, and the family dog. She drove to her parents' home in Dormont. I could not recall for sure that I had seen Mary Regina walk out that particular day, but I had seen her walk out on her own volition before, for breakups after which Dad would go to Dormont to bring her back. Subsequently, Mary Regina would claim that Dad threw her out. I could not picture my father as an aggressor or my mother as a victim. She was hard, and I could not remember ever seeing her shed a tear over anything.

On Tuesday, July 30, on the second business day after Mary Regina left, her lawyer filed her divorce action, starting the 4,900-day era of Beerman-vs-Beerman litigation. I wondered whether the quick filing of the complaint was a sign that it had been prepared in advance and was already set to go when Mary Regina departed from the home.

Chapter 3: Divorce

On August 28, 1968, Mary Regina's first attorney filed a Bill of Particulars, or allegations. On the same day, he filed a petition that counsel fees and costs be paid by Dad.

On March 13, 1969, a different attorney for Mary Regina filed an enhanced "Amended Bill of Particulars."

The Amended Bill of Particulars changed the original claim, "Plaintiff moved out of the Plaintiff and Defendant's home," to "Defendant demanded that the Plaintiff leave their common domicile and find a separate place to reside and provided her with the sum of $100 to leave."

The Amended Bill of particulars also inserted, after "[she was] continually forced to accept charity from her parents and family," the phrase, "for the next 17 years."

Among other embellishments added to the original Bill of Particulars was: "The Defendant on numerous occasions threatened the Plaintiff with physical and/or bodily harm to her person making menacing gestures and intimidating remarks, causing Plaintiff to be in fear and in a constant state of tension and anxiety concerning the possibility of these threats being consummated into acts by the Defendant." I viewed this particular claim as incredible, based on my experience as a resident of the Beerman home.

The Amended Bill of Particulars appears as a supplement at the back of this book.

As outlined earlier in Chapter 1, after a 1-day trial on March 14, 1969, a court-appointed master filed a report saying Mary Regina had not proven her case, and recommended her divorce be denied. Various subsequent lawyers requested delays so they could file exceptions, and ultimately the case was not resolved until a decade later after much legal maneuvering and expense. My vague

Chapter 3: Divorce

understanding was that Mary Regina lost the first case, Dad filed and lost a second case, and finally a "consent order" was filed in January 1982 in which they were declared divorced and Dad was ordered to pay $375 per month in alimony.

A copy of the 1971 master's report appears as a supplement at the back of this book.

No detailed records – only indices of filings – were retrievable from the Allegheny County divorce court for proceedings in the case after 1971.

I assessed that in the Amended Bill of Particulars, Mary Regina and her attorney had wordsmithed and stretched points and complaints to the utmost. I perceived much of it to be "weasel wording."

I believed the litigation should have been put to rest with a "consent order," or settlement, after the first master's recommendation in 1971. With hindsight, it was clear the marriage had been hopeless. However, that might not have been so evident to the Court in the initial years of the litigation. I also believe that logically, anything Dad did after Mary Regina left and filed for divorce should have been deemed irrelevant in legal proceedings. But under the law Dad and Mary Regina were still considered married while separated from 1968 until 1982, and Dad was considered accountable for not being faithful to Mary Regina for those 13 years.

Dad was fortunate that his sister was an employee and friend of a top tier lawyer, Attorney Dennis C. Harrington. Even though Harrington was unable to shorten the long legal process, he did provide a competent, sympathetic, and nonprofit defense, and allowed Dad to work off legal costs

Chapter 3: Divorce

by doing electrical and other jobs at the Harrington home, farm, and cottage. I do not know the details, but I believe Harrington probably advanced court costs on behalf of my financially ruined father. The large Harrington family, including several of their nine children and their long-term house guests, also provided my beleaguered father with much needed friendship.

Harrington was a renowned medical malpractice and personal injury lawyer and a partner in Harrington, Feeney, & Schweers, the law firm that evolved from the P.J. McArdle law firm, which hired Dad's twin Jean after high school in 1943. Harrington's 2009 obituary in the *Pittsburgh Post-Gazette* said, "In his prime ... Mr. Harrington was considered Pittsburgh's premier plaintiffs' lawyer." I doubt that Harrington ever handled a divorce case other than Dad's, unless it was *pro bono* for another needy person.

Harrington had a reputation for competence and integrity. He attended two Catholic Universities – Catholic University in Washington, DC, and Duquesne University in Pittsburgh – and received his law degree from the University of Pittsburgh in 1951. During his career as a trial lawyer with a national reputation, he served as president of the Allegheny County Bar Association, the Pennsylvania Bar Association, and the Allegheny County Academy of Trial Lawyers. He served as chairman of the Pennsylvania State Ethics Commission and the Disciplinary Board of the Supreme Court of Pennsylvania.

I noticed that Harrington had a courtly bearing and charisma. Eyes turned toward him as he entered a courtroom, slowly placed his hat and coat on the rack near the door, and walked through the opening in the railing that

Chapter 3: Divorce

divided the gallery seats from the inner sanctum reserved for officers of the court.

* * *

Mary Regina liked to tell people that my father had thrown her out, and that she and her daughter were "destitute." I didn't doubt that my mother and sister had severe financial limitations. However, I felt that Mary Regina's financial situation was one of her own making. Actually, I wondered whether Dad had worse financial circumstances even though he was the one who had to go to work in a challenging job all through the divorce conflict and he earned what would have been sufficient money in a normal family situation.

Mary Regina moved in with her parents in a modest but nice house in the town of Dormont, where my grandparents had two spare rooms. However, possibly because Mary Regina could not get along with her mother or father, she eventually moved out into the first of two apartments with her daughter.

Dad had all of the bills to pay, including a mortgage, and a burden of court costs.

Dad bore the costs of years of divorce proceedings while Mary Regina was collecting alimony *pendente lite*, or alimony pending the outcome of the case, from him. At the time, as I understood the situation, Pennsylvania did not have alimony, but it had "temporary" alimony *pendente lite,* and that was significant in a case that went on "temporarily" for so long. Of course, Dad also paid child support, which was taken out of his pay.

Mary Regina took a number of actions during the divorce years that did not endear her to me. According to

Chapter 3: Divorce

Dad, she annually reported him to the IRS with allegations of tax evasion. He said she reported him to U.S. Steel headquarters for lying on his job application by claiming falsely that he was a high school graduate. And, Dad said, she also told U.S. Steel headquarters that Dad was stealing company property from the mill.

Mary Regina showed up with her mother at the former family home 364 days – or 1 day short of a year -- after moving out, to spend one night. They sat on the couch all night. This was to comply with a technicality that precluded Dad from claiming she deserted him. I thought this tactic was a travesty, since I believed my mother actually had deserted the home. I wondered why spending the eve of the anniversary of her departure at her former home would legally, logically, or morally make any difference.

On two other occasions, Mary Regina came with someone else, when no one was home. With help, she cumulatively removed virtually all of the contents of the house.

One of Mary Regina's more complicated questionable actions involved the sale of the family home. Dad most likely could not afford to keep up the mortgage payments on the house in Port Vue, or he simply chose to stop. I remember clearly that as the mortgage was going into foreclosure, the local real estate agent came to the front door one day asking for Dad. Dad subsequently told me either that the agent had offered to buy the house for $12,000, or he had offered to list and market it for $12,000.

I could not remember for sure, but I believed the offer probably was to purchase the house. This would be consistent with the practices of some real estate agents in such distressed-sale situations. The goal commonly would

Chapter 3: Divorce

be for the agent to get the owner's signature on a sales agreement at a below-market price, thereby getting control of the property, and then "wholesale" off the sales agreement to another investor, put the house on the market himself, or buy the house himself. In any case, Dad agreed to the agent's offer, which would have been a better alternative for the family than a sheriff sale.

However, Dad said the agent later told him that Mary Regina refused to sign the agreement papers. So, instead of going through with a sale or a sales listing that possibly could have saved more of the equity in the house for the divorce settlement, Mary Regina chose to force the house into a sheriff sale. To me, this seemed to be one of a number of instances of self-harming irrational behavior by Mary Regina.

I later thought it was interesting that the son of one of Mary Regina's longtime good friends, and former next door neighbor, ended up with the house. I thought that one possibility was that Mary Regina simply was trying to do her friend a selfless favor by allowing the friend to buy the house at a bargain price at the sheriff sale. Another possibility was that the neighbor would share the gain inherent in the bargain price with Mary Regina. Of course, a third possibility was that there was no collusion at all. The neighbor simply might have known of the sheriff sale and put in a winning bid.

But the fact remained that Mary Regina had refused to go along with the real estate agent's offer, which forced the sheriff sale and appeared contrary to the best interests of Mary Regina and Dad.

In 2015, I decided to check the Allegheny County records regarding the sheriff sale of the family home. The

Chapter 3: Divorce

records disclosed that almost 3 years after Mary Regina moved out, the sheriff deed for the family home was transferred to the son and daughter-in-law of Mary Regina's friend, for a bid price of $8,400, on June 11, 1971. Thus, the house was sold by the sheriff for $3,600 less than, or only 70 percent of, the $12,000 for which the real estate agent offered to buy it or list it. Probably, the actual market value was even more than $12,000, I thought.

***

Dad truly suffered from the breakup of his marriage and the divorce litigation. I believe he ultimately died young because of it. In other words, I believe my mother drove my father to an early death. One way that Dad suffered was through a bad case of ulcers. In my sixties, I myself had a prolonged acid reflux condition due to a hiatal hernia, so I can appreciate the pain Dad went through with his stomach trouble. Finally, Dad got some relief when the medication Tagamet came on the market in 1979, more than a decade after the start of the divorce proceedings. But even after his ulcers were treated, Dad still suffered great anxiety and hardship.

I remember that during the divorce proceedings, Dad had as his only vehicle for a time a 1950 Chevy with a cracked windshield. It was about 20 years old during the days when cars did not age well. A previous owner had painted the car Navy blue with a paint brush. Mary Regina had the former family car, a 1963 Dodge Dart.

In the days before Tagamet, Dad would drink milkshakes to put out the stomach fires caused by his ulcers. I remember an incident in which Dad had driven me in the '50 Chevy on a winter evening to a soft ice cream shop at the top of Dravosburg Hill, outside McKeesport, to

Chapter 3: Divorce

get milkshakes. When Dad came out of the shop with the milkshakes, the Chevy would not start. Dad had to lie down on the ground in the slushy, muddy unpaved parking lot, shimmy under the car on his back, and struggle with a jammed shift linkage connection to get the car started. Dirty water dripped on him from the underside of the car. Dad, who did not like cold weather, was shivering violently when he finally got the car started.

This incident represented to me the many years of suffering that Dad went through. It also showed me that my father was tough and durable, though not invincible, and that he did not give up when faced with demoralizing problems, especially physical ones such as broken down mechanical equipment that could be fixed with effort and determination. Dad would come to grips with stubborn, rusty, malfunctioning equipment, using his bare hands, even if they were freezing, bruised, cut, and aching.

As professional and amateur mechanics know, mechanic work can be painful as a mechanic strains to reach, and apply force to, a bolt or mechanical component while lying on his or her back or bending over in an awkward position under the hood. The repair person must overcome muscle pain if he or she is to succeed in making the repair. If a wrench slips off a bolt as extreme force is being applied, fingers can be smashed against steel. Some jobs can take hours. Dad could not afford to take his cars to a repair garage, where labor-saving power tools and hydraulic lifts were used. He had to work outside, summer and winter, during rain or snow, often lying on the ground, with whatever tools he happened to have.

Dad bought an upgrade car, a 1957 Oldsmobile that had been sitting in some weeds for a few years. He hoped

Chapter 3: Divorce

that the car, by some miracle, had not incurred damage from being idle for so long.

When Dad got the car started, it spewed smoke. He put additives such as STP in the oil, hoping they would resolve the smoking. He lost his gamble that the car would be okay. It turned out the car's engine had a cracked cylinder head, which could not be repaired for an affordable cost. The engine smoked and steamed and sometimes got so hot that it would vibrate and make a deep humming sound like a church organ. Near the end of the car's short life with the Beermans, Dad let me take it to State College. I carried a few extra gallons of radiator water with me on the 130-mile trip.

I drove the car down College Avenue, which has shops on one side and a hill sloping up to the Penn State campus on the other. The stores and the hill form a shallow valley through which College Avenue passes. I remember looking in the rear view mirror as I drove down College Avenue, and I saw that the gap between the stores and the hillside was filled with steam and smoke from the Oldsmobile's exhaust. Someone commented that the scene looked like a destroyer laying down a smoke screen. I abandoned the car at a repair garage when it broke down on the way home, in the village of Water Street 26 miles from State College. It sat there outside the garage for years and to my knowledge it never ran again.

During the divorce litigation, the money supply was so inadequate that during one particular term at school, I resorted to a diet of tuna sandwiches and popcorn for a time. I could get three sandwiches out of a can of tuna, and I could also fill my belly up cheaply by eating popcorn and drinking water. I worked part time for a while flipping

Chapter 3: Divorce

burgers and cleaning up at a Hardee's hamburger restaurant in State College, and I was able to get some free food there.

I took a classmate from the Journalism Department home with me one weekend in 1969 or 1970. The girl met my father at the Beerman home, which at that time was a messy bachelor house. The three of us went to a flea market on a Saturday.

I wondered what the student had thought of my depressing home environment. I suspected that she told my faculty advisor, Professor William Dulaney, PhD, about my sad home life. Shortly after the visit, the administrative staff at the Journalism Department inexplicably offered me a gratuitous job carrying mail bags up the steps of the Carnegie Building to the Journalism Department office once a day. The job paid a few dollars a week. Dr. Dulaney suddenly seemed to take an interest in my work as a student and he made sure he found me a newspaper job to go to after graduation.

I remember seeing some of the family's possessions -- those not taken by Mary Regina -- be lost when someone came to clean out the garage prior to the sheriff sale. The last vestiges of the worldly possessions from the former family home were thus disposed of. Among the items removed was an inoperable car -- for which I was still making payments -- that I had been storing in the garage. The car was towed away and I never received any money for it. I had to keep making the monthly payments to pay off the car loan anyway.

Such experiences with financial difficulties instilled in me a lifelong sympathy for poor people, especially those who struggle to earn their own living. The hard times also taught me that worldly possessions can come and go, so I

Chapter 3: Divorce

never really cared about such things later in life, although I would not want to see my wife or children lose possessions. My youthful experiences, especially the sheriff sale of the family home, gave me my own personal perspective for the often quoted statement and Thomas Wolfe novel title, *You Can't Go Home Again*.

For much of the time while the divorce proceedings were pending, Mary Regina did not work, and she contended she was unable to do so because of health issues, which was true to a degree. One of her problems was a bout with breast cancer, which resulted in a single mastectomy. But often it seemed she could devote full time to pursuing her vendetta against Dad. Meanwhile, Dad was occupied during most of his waking hours working in the mill, which put him at a disadvantage and on defense in the divorce battle. However, Dad lacked the guile to go on the offense against Mary Regina even if he had had the necessary time.

When looking through Mary Regina's photos after her death, I found one of my father, with notes on the back, that apparently had been provided to a private investigator that Mary Regina or one of her lawyers hired to gather evidence against Dad. The notes were a description of Dad, and said, "5'5-1/2, 140 lbs, 47 age, cig. [cigarette brand] Camel or Pall Mall, pipe, Wm or Bill, droop left shoulder." If he was 47, this would have been written about 3 years after the first divorce trial. Also printed on the back of the photo was an address where a girlfriend of Dad's lived.

***

According to Dad, every year for a number of years, Mary Regina reported him to the IRS, accusing him of tax evasion. He complained that although he was paying my college tuition and living expenses such as rent, the IRS

Chapter 3: Divorce

would not allow him to claim me as a dependent. He said Mary Regina told the IRS that I was working my own way through school. I spent much of the money I earned working in the steel mill during two summers before school resumed in the fall, and rightly or wrongly I did depend on my father for support such as tuition and rent.

Dad told me that because he could not produce canceled checks to equal the required amount to claim a dependent, he could not claim me. As a result, money that could have been retained within the family was being paid instead to the IRS. Furthermore, the need to pay a big IRS bill with penalties and interest when there wasn't enough money for the family's expenses imposed an added psychological strain on Dad.

Dad told me that finally, one day during an audit, he became exasperated with the IRS and vented his frustration at the auditor, complaining that his wife was using the IRS to harass him year after year. Dad said that the auditor, who was a male, expressed interest in the history of the case, checked out Dad's complaint, and finally put an end to the annual audits.

I wondered whether Mary Regina had been collecting rewards from the IRS for turning in Dad.

Other ideas that Mary Regina came up with to "get" Dad involved his job. According to Dad, he was called in by his boss to explain after Mary Regina reported to U.S. Steel headquarters in Pittsburgh that Dad had lied on his job application about having a high school education. Fortunately, Dad's boss, the general foreman, who was named "Berman," apparently believed Dad was a valuable subordinate, so Mr. Berman helped Mr. Beerman get through this problem.

Chapter 3: Divorce

On a separate occasion, according to Dad, Mary Regina reported him to U.S. Steel for stealing equipment from the steel mill. She would sometimes enter the former family home when no one was there and on one such incursion she reportedly saw and took a voltage meter used by Dad on his job. I assumed the meter was marked, "Property of U.S. Steel Corp." Dad said Mary Regina claimed the meter was evidence that Dad was stealing. He explained that he used the meter at home for his job-related self-improvement studies.

These incidents were not considered minor by Dad, and they upset him. Although he managed to avoid getting fired, which apparently was what Mary Regina wanted, traumatic events such as getting called in to his boss's office about lying and stealing, or having his pay attached through court orders delivered to his employer, took a toll on him. Divorce was far less common in those days than it is today, and in the eyes of some people, individuals involved in a divorce wore a stigma of dishonor. The ulcers were a manifestation of Dad's physical suffering, but there was real mental suffering as well.

In my mind, these incidents could not be explained as anything other than the irrational actions of a woman who was bent on destroying her husband, even at the cost of getting him fired from the job that was supporting her as well as him.

Mary Regina seemed to have transformed from the fragile flower of her high school days into a honey badger, reputed to be the meanest and most fearless creature in the animal kingdom. In his book, *The Honey Badger*, author Robert Ruark described the animal as one that "attacks straight for the balls." At times, Mary Regina seemed to personify the quotation that has lived for centuries:

Chapter 3: Divorce

Heaven has no rage like love to hatred turned,
Nor hell a fury like a woman scorned
— English playwright William Congreve
in "The Mourning Bride," 1697

Court records showed that Mary Regina conducted two forays into her former home to remove all of the furniture, carpets, and miscellaneous other items such as the couple's record collection, in January 1971, 30 months after she filed for divorce. As part of one of these incursions, someone dumped the contents of my bedroom furniture into a pile on the floor in the middle of my room, in the process of taking the furniture. I was working in Pittsburgh and living in an apartment in Shadyside at the time, 6 months after graduating from college, and I didn't especially care about the furniture, or even feel that it was mine, although it was from my room.

Dad's lawyer filed a petition with the court to have Dad's share of the home's contents deducted from Mary Regina's *alimony pendite* payments.

In the motion, the attorney wrote:

"That in removing the household furnishings, plaintiff acted with a viciousness and wantonness that is difficult to describe in words. Windows were broken, tables were upset and with force ripped from their attachments, the rugs were removed from the floor, the contents of the refrigerator and shelves were piled in the sink and on the floor."

Photographs were attached.

"That the plaintiff has demonstrated by this and prior acts conduct which is designed to harass and humiliate the defendant in such a way as to prove her hatred for the defendant," the brief asserted.

Chapter 3: Divorce

The motion said Mary Regina removed all of Dad's personal belongings, including the bed in which he was sleeping and the towels and washcloths necessary to maintain personal cleanliness. "The defendant is without the bare essentials necessary to maintain the most humble existence," the motion said.

The petition asked that Dad's court-ordered payments be suspended for 40 weeks so he could purchase furniture and other essentials. I don't know whether the petition was granted.

I believe that among the items taken from the home in an earlier such visit by Mary Regina was a tape recorder that Dad rigged up to record his phone calls. Some reels of tape also were taken. In this instance, Dad's resourcefulness with electronics brought upon him one of his life's most deeply troubling experiences, and certainly aggravated his ulcers.

A considerable time after Mary Regina's departure, as I came to understand it, Dad was involved with a woman. He made some recordings of compromising, lewd, phone conversations between himself and the woman. Mary Regina reportedly captured the recorder and the tapes. I believed Mary Regina, after hearing the tapes, may have played them for Dad's young daughter, my sister, which possibly resulted in her writing the previously mentioned letter in which she called her father a pig.

No reference to tapes was contained in the scarce court records available to me, but I think Dad told me the tapes were played in open court at some point during the years of litigation, adding immeasurably to Dad's burden of stress as he first anticipated, and finally endured, the humiliation.

Chapter 3: Divorce

Dad spoke from the grave with a statement that he was not the despicable man portrayed by Mary Regina to her daughter. He told me by phone one day that he was designating me as one of his two life insurance beneficiaries, along with his second wife, Carol, but he wanted me to share my half equally with my sister, informally. It was a two-sentence discussion. I said okay. Possibly Dad did not want Carol to know he was leaving money to his estranged daughter, because Carol might have thought this was foolish.

After Dad died in 1990, the insurance check came as promised, and Dad was proven true to his word. I dutifully passed half to my sister. I thought that a horrible man who did not care about his daughter, as he was portrayed by Mary Regina, would not arrange to provide his daughter with a gift of insurance proceeds after his death. His motivation was pure; he would not be around to be thanked.

When I told my wife, Martha, about my mother's conduct, she commented that my mother sounded like the mother from the movie *Mrs. Doubtfire*. She was referring to the 1993 film in which Robin Williams played a sympathetic character who is sued for divorce by his wife, Sally Field, and loses custody of his children. I replied that I thought the conduct of the Sally Field character was comparatively benign.

As tough as Mary Regina was in her divorce battle, she would be no match for the challenges she would face later in a nursing home.

Chapter 4: Life After Divorce

I was estranged from my mother and sister for years after the traumatic experiences of the horrible 1968 Christmas visit at my grandparents' house, and the first divorce trial in 1969.

After moving out of the Fishers' home, Mary Regina and Jeanne lived in modest but respectable apartments in Brookline, a borough bordering Dormont, and in Mount Lebanon Township.

There came a time when I made a deliberate decision to renew contact with my mother and sister. I felt that if they were facing hard times, I should do what I could, if anything, to help. I began calling and visiting my mother. On my visits I would do small chores that Mary Regina asked of me such as installing a ceiling fan, shampooing carpets and furniture, or painting her kitchen. I worried a little that my father might consider me disloyal, but he never said anything about it.

I made little money as a newsman and not a lot later as I climbed the pay ladder from GS-9 to GM-14 over 30

Chapter 4: Life After Divorce

years with the Department of Defense. I had to borrow the down payment on my first house from Household Finance Company. I arranged to pick up the loan money 2 hours before the closing on the house purchase, so the loan would not show up on my credit report and jeopardize approval of the mortgage.

The only ways I could accumulate some extra money after paying my bills were to solicit house-painting jobs or work nights in a second job as a newspaper reporter. I accumulated some net worth by improving the homes in which I lived, and making a profit when I sold them. I was limited in what I could do for my mother financially partly because I had the security of my wife and children to think about as my top priority.

At my sister's wedding, I felt like a poor in-law, since my brother-in-law's family was relatively well off. Many years later this feeling would be affirmed. While descending in an elevator in Mary Regina's nursing home after a visit with Mary Regina, in the presence of my brother-in-law and me, my teenage niece commented sadly with a sigh, to no one in particular, "She (Mary Regina) is so poor."

* * *

In 1978 I took a job in Philadelphia and moved to Southern New Jersey, across the Delaware River from Philadelphia.

I bought my mother an old used car from a co-worker in 1980, and made some repairs to it myself. I drove it from New Jersey to Pittsburgh. My mother kept it for a year or two. I never bought a new car myself until 1987, when I was working a second job at the *Philadelphia Inquirer*. This job covered the car payments.

Over the years my mother and I would keep in touch by phone and with visits. We would discuss my sister and her family, Mary Regina's health, and even politics. I brought Mary Regina out to New Jersey about 20 times. She would take a train to Philadelphia or fly economy airlines such as People's Express to Newark, where I would pick her up. While in New Jersey, she could see her grandchildren, William Junior, who lived with me, and Heidi, who lived with her mother near my home. My mother and I would not talk about the unpleasantness of the past. I succeeded in resisting occasional temptations to call her out about her treatment of my father.

At one point, Mary Regina began saying "I love you" at the end of her phone conversations, or as she was departing for a train or flight. I wondered if this was something she picked up from her in-laws, who did that. I would reply in kind, uncomfortably.

I would send my mother money on her birthday, Christmas, and Mother's Day, and would frequently ask her if she needed anything. She always protested that she did not need anything, but she did not hold back in complaining about her health problems. She would remember my birthday, and those of her grandchildren, but not that of my second wife, Martha. After Mary Regina died, I found several checks that I had sent her, still uncashed among her belongings. She had $6,000 in cash in one of two small safes in her bedroom closet.

* * *

Chapter 4: Life After Divorce

I did not talk about the divorce much with my father, either. My father and I remained close. For example, he came to New Jersey to rewire the 75-year-old frame house I bought in Mount Ephraim. It had knob-and-tube wiring and only two glass fuses in the fuse box for the entire house. There was one circuit for the octopus-style boiler, and one for the rest of the house.

Eventually, U.S. Steel started hiring women to work in the mill, and Dad teamed up with one of them. Her name was Carol. He eventually married Carol after the divorce settlement. Combining their incomes, they did okay financially, although they were not without financial difficulties.

I avoided asking Dad for things because I knew he would give me anything I asked for, and I did not want to take advantage of him.

When my first wife, who was pregnant at the time, complained that she was uncomfortable in the summer heat and wished she had a swimming pool, Dad and Carol went out and bought a pool. Dad helped me put it up. Dad and Carol also lavished gifts on the grandchildren, including a bedroom suite with a canopy bed for granddaughter Heidi at the Mount Ephraim house. They took the grandchildren on a number of vacation trips.

McKeesport was in a downward economic spiral during the Seventies and Eighties and much of the city was blighted. Many homes were abandoned. Dad and Carol bought for a low price a large stucco house to live in on what was called Pill Hill. Doctors once lived there before the decline of the city. Dad and Carol became neighbors of another foreman from National Tube and his family.

Chapter 4: Life After Divorce

The couple also bought two or three small investment houses in the city of McKeesport at very low prices. They fixed them up using their own labor, much like some house flippers do today, and they rented them out under the U.S. Department of Housing and Urban Development's (HUD's) Section 8 program. Someone stole the furnace out of one of the rental properties while it was being rehabbed, and I helped Dad replace it with a used one that he bought somewhere.

The McKeesport economy continued to decline, and eventually Dad took an early retirement offer and he and Carol decided to move to Florida. They auctioned their possessions and left a real estate manager to handle the houses in McKeesport. Some street-wise tenants complained to HUD civil servants about minor defects such as broken counterweight chains in a couple of double-hung windows, and HUD allowed Dad's tenants to put their rent payments into escrow pending repairs. Dad, living in Florida, was caught by surprise when HUD returned his rent money to the tenants because of delinquent repairs and he consequently abandoned the properties, just as many other properties were being abandoned in the city.

During his retirement in Florida, Dad repaired boat motors for a friend who owned a marina, and maintained portable traffic signals that controlled traffic during road construction projects on the inter-island roadway through the Keys. Once, when one of his traffic signals malfunctioned, Dad, for some reason, did not find out and did not fix it promptly. As a result, motorists were caught in a monumental traffic jam that extended for miles.

While in the Keys, Dad enjoyed his retirement and hosted visits by his grandchildren, nieces, nephews, and

Chapter 4: Life After Divorce

other relatives. He had a huge pet brown pelican that would hop up into his arms.

Dad was afraid of hurricanes. Some of the islands in the Keys were barely above sea level, and Dad and Carol lived in an Airstream classic travel trailer and kept their Class A-style motorhome parked next to it in a pleasant recreational vehicle and trailer community. The Airstream was fastened down with hurricane cables imbedded in the coral, as required by local building codes. Dad read all the books in the local library about the history of Florida hurricanes, and he and Carol would go north in their motorhome to visit relatives during hurricane season. They also toured parts of the western U.S. and Mexico.

***

Almost everyone seemed to like Mary Regina in her post-divorce life, and she had many friends.

During the Eighties, she lived at an apartment building at 44 Academy Avenue, off Washington Road in Mount Lebanon. She worked 37.5 hours a week for 4 years from 1983 to 1986 for the Pennsylvania Bureau of Employment Security as an unemployment compensation interviewer. She earned about $14,000 a year and an eventual $100-per-month state pension, after a lump sum withdrawal of $3,100 at the time of her retirement in January 1988 at age 62.

The tiny pension, when added to her monthly Social Security benefits of about $1,200, later proved to be the factor that disqualified Mary Regina from potential Medicaid payments for a nursing home in 2011, when she was 86. She had not yet incurred bills for the nursing home care, since Medicare was to pay for the first 100 days.

Chapter 4: Life After Divorce

Eventually the cost of the nursing home, about $9,000 a month, most likely would have been deducted from her income, wiping it out, and it would have made her eligible for Medicaid.

I presumed that Mary Regina's alimony ended with the death of Dad in 1990.

Mary Regina also sometimes worked preparing taxes for H&R Block during tax seasons.

After Jeanne married and Mary Regina retired, Mary Regina moved into a HUD-subsidized senior citizen apartment building, Parkside Manor, in the 1300 Block of Brookline Boulevard, in Brookline, near the border with Dormont.

She then got onto the waiting list for another senior citizen apartment building, Creedmoor Court, which was under reconstruction a short distance away at 1050 Creedmoor Avenue. Creedmoor Court was a pleasant building. It was a high-ceilinged, tastefully decorated and carpeted residence that had been transformed from the multistory former Resurrection Catholic elementary school by a masterful architect. Mary Regina was the first tenant to move in and she got her choice of the one-bedroom apartments. Mary Regina furnished her Creedmoor Court apartment nicely, and hung elegant extra-long heavy draperies on the large windows.

Mary Regina maintained until her death her own independent-living apartment in Creedmoor, which was a Christian Housing, Inc, HUD-subsidized senior citizens building. It was managed by a Catholic nun, and was next door to the Catholic Church of the Resurrection, where Mary Regina attended Mass almost daily.

Chapter 4: Life After Divorce

Mary Regina seemed to be well thought of at Creedmoor Court. She generally made a good impression. She was tallish with a trim figure for her age. She dressed nicely and was articulate. For example, rather than say she was "broke," she would say she was "destitute." Some who knew of her Cathedral High School education may have been impressed with that. She was active socially and did volunteer work for her state representative.

The family of her son-in-law, and Mary Regina's nieces and nephews in Pittsburgh, the offspring of Jack Fisher, loved her. Like the good Catholics they were, the Fishers looked after her and in her later years her nieces would check in on her, take her shopping, and help her clean her apartment.

My Fisher cousins cordially invited me to dinners and to the Fisher family's Fourth of July cookout in 2011 while Mary Regina was in the hospital or the nursing home. After her death, they helped me give away Mary Regina's things, clear out her apartment, and clean it for the next occupant. It didn't require much cleaning. When I thanked the Fishers, they told me that they were happy to do it for Mary Regina's sake.

My mother left behind thousands of photographs of her and her daughter's family having fun on countless vacations and excursions. The pictures showed Mary Regina smiling in scores of activities such as canoeing and hiking. She also took trips with her fellow senior citizens.

In one album, there were photos from trips to Victoria, British Columbia, and Seattle, in 1990; Montana, in 1992; Deer Acres Falls, MI, in 1993; Pyramid Point Trail, MI, in 1994; Mt. St. Helen's, in 1995; Bend, OR, in 1995; Horsetail Falls, OR, in 1996; Southern Oregon, in 1997;

Chapter 4: Life After Divorce

Wisconsin Dells, WI, and Navy Pier, Chicago, in 1999; and Beechwood Resort, Ontario, and Williamsburg, VA, in 2001.

As noted, I wondered whether Mary Regina's personality had been transformed because she became religious or because her thyroid and adrenal gland conditions were ultimately treated successfully. Then again, I recalled, when I was young and living at home, her mood seemed to change instantly from gloomy to cheery if a visitor would come to the house. Maybe my father and I were the only ones with whom she had issues.

I also thought that maybe her personality had changed because of her divorce settlement. Possibly the marriage and the divorce process had been making her ill, and the final consent agreement was the cure.

Nonetheless, after the divorce, there were still strains in the mother-son relationship as the decades wore on. Particularly, Mary Regina would try to impose her will in my parenting of my children. When visiting, Mary Regina would interfere in my child-management efforts although she was unaware of the circumstances with which I was struggling, part of the time as a single parent.

Although my second wife Martha and I had deliberately chosen to buy a house in Haddon Heights, NJ, because it seemed to be an ideal town in which to raise children, several of William Junior's young friends or hockey teammates, and one of Heidi's friends, died in tragic circumstances in separate instances. Those were only the cases I knew about; there could have been more.

Drugs permeating the suburban society in those days were a big concern of mine, and I feared my children would

Chapter 4: Life After Divorce

fall victim to drugs. One day I called the police when I overheard some older boys invite my son to go smoke grass.

I believed it was my responsibility to come to grips with discipline problems even at risk of harming my relationships with my children. The easy way would have been to let things slide, but I felt the proper thing to do was to face the challenges. If my son did not come home on time at night, I would go out and look for him, even though I very much liked to go to bed early.

Mary Regina would take the side of the children, thereby reinforcing their teenage misconceptions that they were right even as they asserted absurd arguments. I resented interference by someone who lacked a factual basis for decision making or for forming opinions, especially someone who had wreaked havoc in her own family.

Fortunately, my two children and the three of my second wife, Martha, all made it into adulthood okay. I attribute this to luck, to my struggles, and to the children for each having a fundamental measure of good sense.

Similarly, Mary Regina had little knowledge about my breakup with my ex-wife, yet, after Mary Regina's death, I found among her things correspondence between her and my "ex" in which they exchanged critical comments about me and commiserated about their respective financial situations.

***

After my sister Jeanne's death, Mary Regina told me she would soon be following her daughter. She was not happy.

Chapter 4: Life After Divorce

Mary Regina said in one phone conversation that although she would do her own shopping, people in the grocery store were beginning to ask her if she was okay. She had COPD (chronic obstructive pulmonary disease) from a lifetime of smoking and shoppers could hear that her breathing was labored.

In late summer 2010 my wife Martha and I visited Mary Regina in Pittsburgh. She told us she wanted to go to the Kennywood amusement park in West Mifflin, PA. She was able to walk around the park and enjoy one or two tame rides. This outing was not only recreational but nostalgic for me and my mother. Kennywood was founded in 1898 and school picnics there were a strong Pittsburgh tradition. Mary Regina and I had gone there annually for our respective school picnics as elementary school children -- she in the Thirties, and I in the Fifties and Sixties.

In May 2011, I made another trip to Pittsburgh to see in person how Mary Regina was doing. I found that she was still able to go out with me. She went with me to rent a rug shampooer at the grocery store. We also went to the office of the local state legislator, to have documents notarized. The documents gave me her medical and financial powers of attorney -- a dubious honor. Then, at her request, we went to her bank to have me replace my deceased sister as co-owner of Mary Regina's checking account.

Mary Regina reviewed many of her papers with me, as we sat on her living room floor amid the contents of two small safes and several accordion folders. She explained her insurance policies, her pre-paid funeral plan, and her burial arrangements. She told me she wanted me to divide certain property, including her cash, equally among her four grandchildren and she specified to whom she wanted

Chapter 4: Life After Divorce

to leave certain furniture. She had no will, but looking back, I concluded she had been quite aware of how her property would be distributed under the law in the absence of a will, in legal terminology, *intestate*.

Mary Regina was lucid during this visit, as always, and she had a firm grasp of all of the circumstances of her affairs – a much better understanding than I could muster myself at that time.

Mary Regina told me a retired nurse who lived in her building was giving her vitamin booster shots. However, Mary Regina seemed to doze off occasionally, and the nurse told me that Mary Regina would soon need some assistance. As usual, when I departed to go back home, I left some money somewhere in the apartment where she would find it, not really believing her claims that she did not need it, and not knowing how much was in her stash of cash.

I began exploring the options for caring for her as she lost her independence, including having her move to New Mexico, or finding an assisted living facility in Pittsburgh.

I arranged for her to visit New Mexico. I flew with her in the spring of 2011 on her trip to New Mexico and I also escorted her on her return flight to Pittsburgh. At Greater Pittsburgh Airport, after a grueling wait standing in the long security-check line, the 85-year-old Mary Regina was pulled aside and given a special security search after she concealed two cigarette lighters in her waist band. Asked why she did not disclose the lighters, she responded, "They would have taken them." (Mary Regina's smoking habit actually caused her to miss a flight on a different occasion because she had gone outside to have a smoke.)

Chapter 4: Life After Divorce

I explained to Mary Regina that she could take an apartment in a nice HUD senior citizen building such as Mira Vista Villas in Las Cruces, or in a regular apartment building such as Regency Pointe in Las Cruces. I told her she was very welcome to live with me and Martha at our home, which was a single-story three-bedroom house with no steps and a nearly level sidewalk. I installed a grab bar in a shower for her during her visit.

I explained that if she wanted privacy, she could have her own place, near our house, and we could help her clean and shop. Or if she wished, she could stay at our home, keeping the apartment as well so she could have a retreat of her own. She would have the best of both worlds. And she could say goodbye to harsh Pittsburgh winters. I thought this would be a splendid arrangement.

I pointed out that my home was within 1 mile of two different hospitals, and that I could recommend my own doctor, who was a specialist in geriatric medicine.

Mary Regina declined repeated offers during her stay in Las Cruces to look at additional potential residences besides Mira Vista Villas and Regency Pointe, and instead snoozed in a chair, watched her favorite TV shows about house flipping, or went to the mall with Martha. She made a remark that the apartments Martha and I showed her were "the projects." I was shocked, and thought the complexes were nice. I was sure that no one else would agree with Mary Regina's characterization of them. She also said she did not want to leave Pittsburgh.

I suspected she did not trust me, which would be understandable given our history. However, I had good intentions. Nevertheless, it had become clear that the best

Chapter 4: Life After Divorce

arrangement in my view -- her coming to New Mexico -- was not an option.

I consulted with A Place for Mom, a service for families looking for living facilities for a parent, about assisted living apartments in Pittsburgh. Eldercare advisor Dave Grimm provided useful lists and helpful advice. For example, he told me about the Aid and Attendance Benefit of $1,149 a month that the surviving spouse of a wartime veteran can put toward his or her home care, nursing home, assisted living community, or personal care. Unfortunately, after learning about the circumstances, Grimm had to point out that when a spouse divorces a veteran, he or she divorces the veteran's benefits too.

One of the assisted living facilities to which Grimm referred me was Devonshire of Mount Lebanon, which was located across McNeilly Road from Keystone Oaks High School, where Jeanne graduated, and a mile up the road from where Mary Regina's brother Jack lived. It also was close to Mary Regina's apartment building, Creedmoor Court, where some of Mary Regina's friends lived. Devonshire was secluded amid nicely landscaped acreage, and the interior of the building was tasteful. The lobby and dining room were hotel-like.

Monthly rates at Devonshire were roughly $3,000 for an efficiency apartment with an assisted living arrangement that included meals and limited nursing support. The manager offered me an independent living arrangement in a one-bedroom apartment for $1,929 a month. It included two meals daily, free transportation, housekeeping, utilities, cable TV, and daily activities. He said that if Mary Regina were to move in with an independent living deal, Devonshire staff could informally check in on her each day to see how she was doing, and make observations such as

Chapter 4: Life After Divorce

whether Mary Regina was taking her medication on schedule.

The manager said the staff would try to maintain Mary Regina's independent living status as long as possible, by providing courtesies such as the medication check. She could later transition to assisted living accommodations as necessary. I had tentatively decided to strongly recommend Devonshire to Mary Regina, when she broke her hip and it eventually became evident that she might, at least temporarily, need a nursing home rather than an independent living or assisted living facility.

The cost of Devonshire's independent living arrangement would have exceeded Mary Regina's income by about $700 a month, or $8,400 a year, so I would have had to subsidize her rent. Mary Regina's son-in-law generously offered to split the subsidy with me.

I regretted that my mother had frustrated my effort during 2002 to enroll her as an eligible family member in a long-term-care insurance policy through the federal employee group program while I was working for the government. My sister Jeanne and I had agreed to split the monthly premiums. However, when Mary Regina filled out the application, she painstakingly portrayed all of her medical conditions so deleteriously that her application was rejected.

Jeanne told me that Mary Regina's doctor had expressed surprise at the rejection and offered to challenge it as inappropriate in a letter to the insurance company or to the Office of Personnel Management. I believed that since the program was a group policy that was being newly initiated for federal employees and their parents, no one should have been rejected for preexisting conditions. But

Chapter 4: Life After Divorce

Mary Regina would not pursue the matter. If Mary Regina had gotten the policy when I applied in 2002, my sister and I would have made at least 9 years of payments before using the policy, and Mary Regina may have never used it, considering when and how she died. This implies that Mary Regina wasn't such a bad risk.

While I was working on the project of making arrangements for my mother, on June 30, 2011, I got a phone call from a cousin telling me that after awakening from a nap, Mary Regina had tripped over a footstool in her apartment, and had broken her left hip and wrist. The manager of Creedmoor Court accompanied Mary Regina to Mercy Hospital (University of Pittsburgh Medical Center (UPMC Mercy)) after the accident.

PART TWO: Hospitals, the Nursing Home, and a Funeral Home

Be nice to your children. After all, they are going to choose your nursing home.
—Comedian Steven Wright

Chapter 5: A Broken Hip and Wrist, and Mercy Hospital

After learning of my mother's fall, I put my affairs in New Mexico in order as quickly as I could and took the first reasonably priced flight to Pittsburgh. It took me several days, including one day of travel time, to get to Pittsburgh. In the meantime, my cousins, the Fishers, looked after Mary Regina.

Chapter 5: A Broken Hip and Wrist

I felt Mary Regina was in good hands at Mercy Hospital, and there was little I could do if I were there. Mary Regina had been hospitalized in the past without me being present, or even knowing about it. Mercy, a Catholic hospital, was founded in 1847, and my mother's family had used it for generations.

I didn't think it was prudent to spend hundreds of extra dollars on a same-day flight and rental car, and at the same time leave loose ends at home. For example, I needed to repair my automatic irrigation system before I left or the July sun and 105-degree temperatures would destroy my lawn and landscaping within 3 or 4 days. I also needed to repair a small spot in the roof that might leak in the rare event of a desert rainstorm.

Upon my arrival at the hospital, I found that Mary Regina was recovering from hip repair surgery and two of my cousins were with her. Mary Regina asked me, "Where were you?" What she meant was, "You sure took your time getting here."

This touched a nerve in me, because I always felt a little sheepish around relatives from my mother's side of the family. I assumed they probably thought I had not been a good son, since they did not know about some of the internal family history or have my perspective on the relationship between my mother and me. I knew that Mary Regina had displayed one personality to outsiders and a different one toward me. But I ignored Mary Regina's question, and said hello to my cousins. They helped dispel the uncomfortable atmosphere with conversation.

The surgery had gone well. The hip, which was broken at the neck of the femur, had been repaired with a Synthes

Chapter 5: A Broken Hip and Wrist

trochanteric nail and locking devices. The wrist was in a short cast.

I stayed that night at Mary Regina's apartment, and I called her from the apartment the next morning before going back to the hospital. She sounded groggy on the phone and asked me, in slurred speech, "Where are you?" Then she asked, "Why don't you stand up and be a man?"

She also said on the phone that during the previous night she was chained to a bed in the basement of St. Clair Hospital -- a different hospital 8 miles from Mercy. "I am in the hospital somewhere, not in my room. Once you look at me you'll know I'm not crazy," she said.

Later, a doctor told me that the effects of anesthesia were lingering and that it took a long time for some elderly patients to completely purge anesthesia from their systems and clear their heads. Sometimes it took days, sometimes weeks, and sometimes the patient never completely returned to normal, the doctor said.

Hospital personnel had Mary Regina stand up next to the bed the day after surgery. Apparently the surgical repair enabled her hip to bear weight.

A nurse told me that the hospital could move Mary Regina to its own in-house rehabilitation therapy floor if she was able to undergo 3 hours of therapy per day. This was not as demanding as it sounded. It did not mean 3 hours of physical therapy, but the 3 hours included "occupational therapy" -- instruction in how to adapt self-care activities like dressing and grooming while recovering from movement-restricting injuries such as the broken wrist and hip. But neither I nor my mother knew that then. I secretly thought 3 hours of therapy sounded challenging.

Chapter 5: A Broken Hip and Wrist

A nurse commented that the hospital would give Mary Regina a blood transfusion to build up her strength for the therapy.

When Mary Regina heard the nurse say "blood transfusion," she raised a fuss. She told the nurse the hospital was not going to give her a transfusion. "I have had many things (medical conditions) worse than this and I've never had a transfusion in my life," she said. "I am not going to have one now." I wondered why she felt so strongly about it, but I never asked and she never told me.

The refusal of the transfusion proved to be a fateful, and fatal, decision. I later wondered whether the transfusion might have helped clear Mary Regina's head of the effects of the anesthesia more quickly, as well as make her stronger.

The next day, July 4, 2011, I was informed that Mary Regina was being discharged from Mercy and she would have to be moved to a nursing home/rehabilitation facility because she did not meet the criteria to remain for inpatient rehabilitation at Mercy. I was certain Mary Regina's obdurate refusal of the transfusion was the critical factor in the decision to move her out. Although I did not realize it then, the transfer decision meant that Mary Regina would not undergo rehabilitation in a vibrant, resource-rich, full-service, fully equipped hospital, with top notch medical personnel on duty 24 hours a day, 7 days a week. Instead, she would go to a below average nursing home that rarely had even a single doctor present onsite, and was sluggish at best in providing care.

I did not know what to do and hospital staff were not much help in accomplishing what should have been a carefully considered transfer to a nursing home that was

Chapter 5: A Broken Hip and Wrist

appropriate for Mary Regina. Hospital personnel whom I asked said they were not permitted to recommend a nursing home.

After two requests from me, the staff at the nurse's station provided me with two computer-printout lists of names and addresses of nursing homes, with basic information such as contact persons and the types of payment accepted. There were 14 nursing homes on each list. They all seemed to accept Medicare and Medicaid. As I had requested, one list had nursing homes in the South Hills area and the other had nursing homes in the east suburbs. There were no ratings on the lists. I learned from someone that because Mary Regina had been hospitalized for 3 days for actual treatment and not just observation, Medicare would cover up to the first 100 days of rehabilitation in a nursing home, as long as she was making progress. ("Actual treatment" and "Making progress" may no longer be requirements today.)

Hospital personnel said they preferred that Mary Regina be transferred out the same day, or the next day at the latest. I told them my mother was not herself because of the anesthesia and I did not think she should be released. I was told I could fill out papers to appeal the release. I chose not to do so partly because I was afraid the medical insurance would not cover the hospital bills if I refused to move Mary Regina after the hospital had discharged her. If I had known what the future held, I would have appealed the release, and I decided later that not appealing the release had been another fatal mistake.

The situation was complicated by my uncertainty about how strongly I should be asserting myself on behalf of my mother, despite the fact that I had her medical power of attorney. Before undergoing the anesthesia Mary Regina

Chapter 5: A Broken Hip and Wrist

had been capable of making her own decisions. And she certainly had made her own decision about the transfusion.

Later, in 2016, I found out that the Centers for Medicare & Medicaid Services (CMS) approved a form (CMS-R-193) in July 2010, entitled, "An important Message from Medicare About Your Rights." It states, "If you think you are being discharged too soon," and you notify the appropriate personnel no later than your planned discharge date and before you leave the hospital, "you will not have to pay for the services you receive during the appeal (except for charges like copays and deductibles)."

It is within the realm of possibility that I was told this. I cannot remember. But I reasoned that I probably had not been made aware fully of the situation, because I doubted that I would have failed to appeal the release if I had known my mother would have been covered by Medicare during the appeal.

Using the list of nursing homes provided by Mercy, my cousin Ellen Fisher and I each drove out separately on July 5 to visit nursing homes on the list. Ellen took two on the eastern side of Pittsburgh, where she lived, since she wanted to be able to visit Mary Regina frequently, and I took two on the southwestern side of town, where other cousins lived and where Mary Regina's apartment building was located. I still had hope of her returning to her apartment at Creedmoor Court after a rehab stay in the nursing home, and I thought Creedmoor residents, some of whom had cars, might visit her at the nursing home.

In retrospect, the process of driving around the county looking at nursing homes from a sample of 28 homes on two lists, with a 1-day deadline, was absurd. Any reasonable person faced with such a task would first try to

Chapter 5: A Broken Hip and Wrist

prioritize the list, but I had no basis for ranking the nursing homes.

I was stressed as I tried to find a nursing home. I had to waste time driving considerable distances in congested traffic and I did not have a GPS (global positioning system) device to help me find the nursing homes.

I did not know how the process worked. I was not even sure any nursing home I selected would accept my mother. If it did, how would she get there? Could I drive her? Would I have to arrange an ambulance? Would I have to pay up front?

The first facility from the Mercy Hospital printout that I visited in the South Hills had the infamous smell of urine even at the front entrance. The second, in the upscale suburb of Upper St. Clair, seemed almost like a plush resort hotel, with the patients dressed up accordingly. At this time, cost was no object because I believed that Medicare and my mother's AARP policy would pay the cost for up to the first 100 days. However, I did not think my mother would be happy in a swanky nursing home for rich people.

Because of legal considerations, the name of the nursing home that I selected is not used in this book. Instead, the nursing home is called Mary Regina's nursing home (MRNH). The conditions I found there are accurately reported.

I do not consider the name of the nursing home to be important because, based on my research and the nursing home's rating, it most likely was similar to many nursing homes with similar ratings in similar nursing home chains across the U.S. However, readers should not necessarily assume the exact conditions prevailing at MRNH exist at

Chapter 5: A Broken Hip and Wrist

those with similar ratings today. Conditions at nursing homes change over time, ratings move up and down, and nursing home ownership changes. Even the rating system changes. So, ratings from one period of time are not necessarily comparable to ratings from another period.

I selected MRNH because it was close to my cousin Ellen's home and she planned to visit my mother often. Also, Ellen believed someone she knew had stayed there and found it to be fine. MRNH did look fine on first impression. I was relieved that MRNH accepted Mary Regina.

Mercy Hospital called MRNH and arranged to have Mary Regina transferred there by wheel-chair van. No one asked for any money.

I drove separately in my rental car as a van transported my mother to MRNH on July 6, 2011.

Sometime after Mary Regina was admitted to MRNH, after it was too late, I went on line to Medicare.gov with my laptop and was surprised to learn that the government rated nursing homes. I had not expected the government would be so frank and critical of private businesses. However, I did not understand then that Medicare and/or Medicaid payments were the financial life's blood of most nursing homes. The federal government, through CMS, wielded federal regulatory power as well as financial power over nursing homes, as did state regulatory agencies, and the government could fine nursing homes or stop their government payments.

I saw that MRNH had an overall rating of only two out of a possible five stars. I was sorry to see the sub-average rating, because it meant I had mismanaged my mother's

Chapter 5: A Broken Hip and Wrist

placement. Another nursing home, a Golden Living Center, located only 3 minutes, or 1 mile from MRNH, had a rating of four stars. One might infer that four stars is twice as good as two. Actually, according to CMS, one star meant much below average, two stars meant below average, three average, four above average, and five much above average.

I eventually concluded, after trying to move Mary Regina out of MRNH, that generally, Catholic nursing homes – such as Little Sisters of the Poor, which I learned later would have been Mary Regina's first choice -- were among a handful in the Pittsburgh area that had five-star ratings. However, the five-star homes had waiting lists. I cynically wondered whether the Catholic facilities with waiting lists gave preference to patients who were financially well off and who might leave large bequests to the nursing homes. I had no evidence to justify such a suspicion, and it was unfair to think that. Nevertheless, as I tried unsuccessfully to move my mother out of MRNH, and became frustrated, the thought went through my troubled mind.

I believed that Mercy Hospital should not have rushed me to transfer Mary Regina out, and should have informed me that Medicare had nursing home ratings on its website. A doctor at Mercy told me that because my mother was discharged over the Fourth of July holiday, some of the "preventive" steps normally followed by the hospital in its discharge process had not been taken.

Later, while going through my mother's medical records, I found a Mercy Hospital doctor's report that stated that because Mary Regina had medical complexities, she required 24-hour availability of a physician and nursing with skilled services that are diverse and complex. Mercy Hospital's own rehabilitation facility fit those criteria.

Chapter 5: A Broken Hip and Wrist

A hospital doctor wrote: "The patient demonstrates the potential for significant practical improvement. The following **acute inpatient** rehabilitation is recommended...."

"Due to the functional impairments and medical complexity, this patient requires provision of rehabilitation services in a setting providing twenty-four-hour availability of a physician with special training in the field of rehabilitation. In addition, the patient will require twenty-four-hour availability of a registered nurse with training and experience in rehabilitation and skilled services which are diverse and complex requiring a coordinated interdisciplinary approach. The patient's condition requires skilled therapy intervention for at least 3 hours per day, 5 days a week, with specific therapies provided...."

"Provision of services in a less intensive environment risks significant complications and a more limited potential outcome."

Yet Mercy released Mary Regina not to an **acute inpatient** facility (which could be interpreted to mean a hospital's in-house rehabilitation facility), but to a below average nursing home (two of five stars in the overall Medicare.gov rating) – a facility that told patients and their families that the nursing home was required by law to call in a doctor only once a month. Technically, a doctor might have been "available" to be called in at the nursing home, but not available onsite to the degree a doctor -- and other medical personnel -- would be available in a hospital. But I did not obtain a copy of the physician's report quoted above, or any other medical records, until after Mary Regina had died.

Chapter 5: A Broken Hip and Wrist

Mary Regina's condition when she left Mercy Hospital was wonderful compared to what it would be when she left MRNH after 21 days there. Mercy Hospital reports portrayed her as being in generally good condition. The transitory confusion attributed to the anesthesia cleared up substantially, although not completely.

One Mercy Hospital report began, "This is a pleasant 86-year-old female...." Another said "Pt. (Patient) is an excellent candidate for rehab." A "Review of Systems" on July 3 said: Constitutional: no fever, no chills, no sweats; Respiratory: no shortness of breath; Cardiovascular: no chest pain; Gastrointestinal: No nausea, No vomiting; Musculoskeletal: No joint pain, No muscle pain. All other systems are negative.

Regarding neurologic, a report said: (Cognitive/Language) Oriented to self, being in hospital, name of hospital, city, year; (Commands) ability to follow simple commands; ability to follow multiple step commands; (Language/speech) fluent; (Sensory) sensory intact to light touch.

Mercy Hospital had been Mary Regina's hospital of choice for virtually her entire life after she left our home in Port Vue, PA. She had also had the same doctor for decades. Her doctor was the son of a close friend, and Mary Regina had helped the doctor move his things when he enrolled in medical school. That doctor was affiliated with Mercy Hospital. But after Mary Regina was sent to MRNH, personnel there told me that her doctor had "no authority here."

Because of my lack of knowledge about the nursing home oversight system and resident advocacy

Chapter 5: A Broken Hip and Wrist

organizations, Mary Regina, with her broken hip and wrist, and I, were on our own.

Chapter 6: Mary Regina's Skilled Nursing Home

On Wednesday, July 6, 2011, I was waiting in the sunshine outside MRNH when a van pulled up with my mother. As she was shown inside by an attendant pushing her wheelchair, I tried to make reassuring comments. Neither I nor my mother had any reason to suspect on that bright summer day that Mary Regina was beginning the last 32 days of her life. But on July 27 she would be loaded into an ambulance outside MRNH and taken away to a hospital emergency room, and by August 7, she would be dead.

A hospital report said that on July 27 Mary Regina became unresponsive and could not be roused at MRNH. Shortly after the ambulance left MRNH with Mary Regina and headed for Mercy Hospital, which is about 12 miles down the Parkway from MRNH, the emergency medical technicians (EMTs) diverted the ambulance to Forbes Regional Hospital. According to MRNH records, the EMTs veered off to the closer hospital because Mary Regina was suffering in the ambulance from dropping oxygen saturation in her blood and difficulty breathing.

Chapter 6: The Skilled Nursing Facility

I thought my mother must have been in critically bad shape when MRNH called the EMTs. MRNH records about the decision to send her to the hospital show she had a "change in mental status," a urinary tract infection, symptoms of dehydration, and blood in her stool. Records show these were not her only medical problems at MRNH.

* * *

When Mary Regina checked in, MRNH was a reasonably attractive building with brick facades. It stood in a pleasant suburban garden-apartment district with lots of greenery.

Inside, MRNH had a counter and desk staffed with a receptionist to assist visitors and ensure they signed a log book and entered their time of arrival, before going inside, and that they signed again, and entered the time, when leaving. The receptionist would phone inside if a visitor asked to see a staff member, and the staffer then would come to the reception area.

There was a couch and some other furniture. A binder containing the results of inspections and surveys done by the Pennsylvania Department of Health lay inconspicuously on an end table. The reception area was separated from the rest of the building by a set of double doors.

MRNH's public area did not smell of urine.

The appearance of the MRNH reception area gave no clue that MRNH was a below average nursing home when Mary Regina and I arrived there. The substandard performance of MRNH would become evident to us later.

MRNH was a for-profit operation with more than 100 beds. According to its website, when I checked years later

Chapter 6: The Skilled Nursing Facility

in December 2015, MRNH, Inc. had a nationwide network of hundreds of skilled nursing and rehabilitation centers, assisted living facilities, outpatient rehabilitation clinics, and hospice and home health care agencies. The majority of these were listed under several different names. MRNH, Inc. had tens of thousands of employees, a substantial portion of whom had been with the company at least 5 years.

A search for the real corporate name of MRNH in Pennsylvania on the Medicare.gov, Nursing Home Compare, Five-Star Rating System website in February 2016 turned up dozens of facilities. In Pennsylvania, 14 percent of MRNH facilities had five stars, 17 percent had four, 21 percent had three, 31 percent had two, and 17 percent had one. For comparison, a search for nursing facilities belonging to another nursing home corporation, Golden Living, in Pennsylvania, turned up 36: two with five stars (6 percent), seven with four (19 percent), 10 with three (28 percent), seven with two (19 percent), and 10 with one (28 percent).

According to my count, 48 percent of the homes in Pennsylvania in the MRNH chain were below average (one or two stars) in the Five-Star ratings system as were 47 percent of those in the Golden Living chain.

Upon admission to MRNH, at 2:15 p.m. on July 6th, Mary Regina was taken in a wheel chair through the double doors, behind which were physical therapy facilities, a kitchen, and some patient rooms, along a hallway. She was given a very brief interview by a MRNH doctor. He wore a wrinkled suit and he did not look to me as if he would have had much of a chance of getting hired if he were to show up at a job interview looking as he did. (To be fair, I must

Chapter 6: The Skilled Nursing Facility

say that later, I met a different MRNH doctor who made a much more favorable impression.)

The rumpled doctor conducted his interview in the hallway, causing me to wonder why the meeting was not held in an office or examining room setting, or in Mary Regina's room.

As I remember it, there were no warm and respectful business-client pleasantries exchanged. The doctor seemed to be impatient and he cut Mary Regina short when she attempted to explain medication issues such as her allergy to penicillin and the fact that she did not want to be given too much pain medication.

Anesthesia from the hip operation still had not worn off entirely and Mary Regina was coherent but not as mentally quick as usual. I thought that if she had not been a little under the influence of anesthesia, her demeanor might have elicited a little more respect from the doctor. The after-effects of the anesthesia obscured some of Mary Regina's personal dignity. Even after the anesthesia dissipated, she would not receive the same deference and courtesy during her residency at MRNH that most businesses would extend to their clients.

Mary Regina's discharge orders from Mercy Hospital called for Tylenol 3 (Tylenol with codeine) for pain, but the MRNH doctor discontinued the Tylenol and prescribed morphine doses of 10 mg PO (by mouth) Q8 (at 8-hour intervals). Later, on the morning of July 13, in response to family concerns expressed repeatedly to the nurses that the medication was too much for Mary Regina, the doctor reduced it to 5 mg, PO TID (3 times per day) PRN, with PRN meaning "as needed," or in other words, as requested.

Chapter 6: The Skilled Nursing Facility

Morphine was not the only drug Mary Regina was being given.

In a documented pain assessment done by MRNH on July 8, Mary Regina rated her present pain on a 10-point scale as zero, her pain at worst as three, and her pain at best as zero. She did, however, rate the frequency of pain as "frequently," according to the assessment document. As a benchmark, a five meant "moderate pain but patient is able to function and interact with environment."

I recalled that the intake "interview" lasted only 5 minutes or so. I later found that some interview notes that I believe the doctor had scrawled during the intake interview were nearly undecipherable to me.

After the interview, Mary Regina was taken in a wheelchair to a room, which had one other patient, similar to a semiprivate hospital room, and she was put into bed. I conversed with Mary Regina's roommate, who seemed happy to have someone to talk to. I was hoping that Mary Regina would join in and warm up to the woman, who was quite congenial. But Mary Regina chose to keep the exchange to a minimum.

Shortly thereafter, dinner arrived.

It was wieners and beans.

A staffer explained that the big meal of the day had been lunch. The next day at lunchtime, a staffer brought a chicken sandwich that Mary Regina did not eat. The second-day dinner was a steak sandwich soaking in a plate of water. Apparently when the kitchen worker spooned a vegetable onto the plate, he or she did not use a slotted spoon to drain off the water, and the water from the vegetable had literally dissolved the bread of the sandwich,

Chapter 6: The Skilled Nursing Facility

making for an unappetizing presentation. Mary Regina did not eat her first four meals at MRNH, according to my notes. She would miss many more meals as the weeks went by.

I knew that the initial meals made a strong, negative, first impression on Mary Regina, who had been getting first class food such as roast beef, mashed potatoes, and gravy at Mercy Hospital. MRNH staff showed no apparent interest in what Mary Regina was eating. I read in the book, *Eldercare for Dummies*, by Rachelle Zukerman, that whether staff assisted patients in eating was an indicator of nursing home quality. Later, when I complained about my mother not eating at MRNH, a staffer, a dietician, said she would order a supplementary diet. That turned out to be the regular diet with a half-pint carton of a supplemental drink added to the tray.

Unfortunately, over the course of her stay, Mary Regina would often be "zonked" (a term used by some nursing home staff), or drugged, at mealtimes, and the staff members would not even leave her tray in the room. They would look in, see her asleep, or in my layman's assessment, unconscious, sometimes with her mouth open, and they would walk away, continuing on down the hall. I thought they should have left the tray, in case Mary Regina woke up. Or ideally, they would have tried to awaken her and coax her to eat. Later, I would read in nursing home records that these walk-bys with the meal trays were described as Mary Regina "refusing" meals. Being cynical, I wondered whether the staff members ate the "refused" meals.

Eventually, on evenings after dinner when Mary Regina was awake, I would sometimes bring her a hamburger, French fries, and a milkshake from McDonalds,

Chapter 6: The Skilled Nursing Facility

or an ice cream sundae from a King's restaurant, where I would go to eat.

I spent virtually every day with Mary Regina during her 3 weeks at MRNH, and my cousin, Ellen Fisher, who was Mary Regina's god-daughter, and other relatives, would visit. Mary Regina's son-in-law and her teenage grandchildren would also come from Michigan to see her, and stay with their relatives near Pittsburgh.

No orientation was provided to Mary Regina as a new patient during her first 48 hours at MRNH. She was given no idea what to expect regarding meals, or anything else. For example, Mary Regina and I were not told she could request an alternative meal by calling the kitchen before a scheduled meal. (Of course, what she actually needed was a chance for a different meal <u>after</u> an unappealing one was delivered.) The lack of a welcome made me wonder what we had gotten into, although I initially hid my concerns from my mother. I did not want to create or aggravate a negative attitude.

Finally, late in the afternoon on July 8, a staff member visited and asked Mary Regina to sign papers. This visitor also provided basic orientation information that mainly pertained to business matters. Mary Regina was drugged at the time she signed the papers, and although her handwriting normally was beautiful, the best she could manage was to make scrawls that were nowhere near the signature spaces on the papers. Later, when I asked MRNH for my mother's records, these papers were not among the records provided.

Mary Regina had periods of lucidity as the days went on, at times when she was not "zonked." I was impressed when I listened in on one side of a phone conversation that

Chapter 6: The Skilled Nursing Facility

Mary Regina had with her son-in-law, who at that time was her daughter's widower. He wanted to bring Mary Regina out to Michigan to live so she could be near him and her grandchildren. In the phone conversation, Mary Regina presented a half dozen compelling arguments about why that would not be a good idea. These included the fact that her son-in-law traveled a lot for business, the fact that her grandchildren were about to go away to college, and the fact that her son-in-law was engaged and about to start a new life with his fiancée. Mary Regina also said she did not want to leave Pittsburgh.

I concluded that her comments on the phone demonstrated strong reasoning power and an ability to articulate her thoughts cogently.

I would try to convince the staff that my mother was being over-drugged and mentally suppressed. Sometimes nursing home personnel would write in the records that she exhibited some confusion. This was exasperating to me. I thought it was as ludicrous for them to say she was confused as it was for them to write in the records that she "refused" meals while she was zonked on drugs and lying unaware that an aide had walked past her door with a food tray.

Mary Regina asked me to bring her certain items of clothing from her apartment in Brookline, where I was staying at night, and she sent me out shopping for other items, such as a Cricket phone. Mary Regina was not helped with dressing, or with grooming during her first 2 days. Because of her broken left hip and with her broken left wrist in a cast, she could not get out of bed on her own without much difficulty, and it would have been risky for her to try. I helped her out twice but I usually went down the hall to the nurse's station to ask that someone help

Chapter 6: The Skilled Nursing Facility

Mary Regina to the bathroom. Later, the physical therapists would come in the morning to help with dressing and grooming as part of occupational therapy. Medicare was billed for this.

I began to realize that more bad signs about MRNH were accumulating.

In the hallway outside Mary Regina's room, an electronic chime rang almost incessantly. As I remember, it seemed to be ringing at least 50 minutes out of each hour during the day. The chime was the alert device that sounded when a patient requested help by pressing a bedside button. The almost unrelenting chime annoyed Mary Regina, who complained about it. She wanted me to walk down to the nurses' station and get the problem solved. It was like the drip, drip, drip of Chinese water torture. But I felt nothing could be done about the chime because it was only a symptom of the staff's failure to respond in a timely manner to requests for patient assistance. The response time would have to be improved to calm down the chime.

Even worse, patients two or three rooms down the hall sometimes would cry out over and over with pleas such as, "Nurse. Nurse. Please help me. Nurse!" and this would go on for what seemed to be 20 or 30 minutes per incident. I initially wondered whether the nurses or aides were ignoring these people because they were known to be malingerers "crying wolf."

After talking with a younger, mentally and generally physically fit patient who was at MRNH only for physical rehabilitation of a relatively minor injury, I concluded MRNH did not deserve the benefit of the doubt. The patient told me he was not pleased with the staff, and he had even

Chapter 6: The Skilled Nursing Facility

experienced rough treatment. During my conversation with this patient, a staffer came jive-stepping down the hallway swinging her arm and singing to herself. She had an air of unfriendliness approaching subtle insolence. After the staffer had passed by, the other patient and I silently communicated our shared displeasure with this unprofessional, inappropriate conduct with an exchange of frowns.

I was caught in a dilemma with my mother complaining about the chime on one hand, and on the other my caution about annoying the staff with complaints about something that was not likely to be corrected anyway.

After hearing the cries coming out of the rooms on several occasions over a period of days, I decided this situation was very wrong and I tried to record the cries with my phone, but I didn't know how to operate the recorder in my phone and I didn't want to be seen trying to record the crying. So, I gave up.

Notes that I prepared in advance of a meeting that I requested with a MRNH representative show I did complain to the staff member at the meeting that: "Bells ring incessantly. Apparent very slow response to calls."

After I found out about the Medicare Five-Star nursing home rating system, when Mary Regina had already been at MRNH for some time, I printed the pertinent ratings from Medicare.gov on July 11, 2011 at the local library. As noted, MRNH had only a two-star overall rating on the five-star scale. Its rating in the subcategory of staffing was also two stars. I was surprised that the rating for staffing was not lower.

Chapter 6: The Skilled Nursing Facility

MRNH did not seem to devote much attention to the residents, aside from responding sluggishly to the nurse-call buttons and verbal calls. Mary Regina repeatedly sent me down to the nurses' station for needs such as water and ice. She needed the ice to treat swelling in her broken wrist. Or, she would ask me to bring someone to help her shift her position in the bed, because she would gradually slide down because of the raised angle of the mattress. She was concerned that her broken wrist and her heels should be kept elevated, as a doctor had ordered.

(Later, when Mary Regina was admitted to Forbes Regional Hospital, staff there reported that her hand was swollen, blue, and cold to the touch. They cut open the cast to relieve the pressure. The Forbes staff told me about this on the telephone and later I found notes about it in the records. The wrist had been re-cast on July 25 by an orthopedic surgeon – 2 days before MRNH sent Mary Regina to Forbes and Forbes personnel cut the cast.)

Mary Regina complained one day that the MRNH staff had treated her roughly during the night, and "threw me around like a sack of potatoes." A subsequent note in her records said a doctor requested that the staff be gentle with her, and that therapists go easy if she was exhausted.

Whenever I would go to the nurses' station with inquiries or requests, the nurse in charge sitting there would be slow to look up, not so subtly making me feel that I wasn't welcome at the desk.

The main problem was over- and under-medicating. On Mary Regina's second or third day at MRNH, when walking by the nurses' station, I heard a nurse on the telephone say, "The problem with Regina Beerman...." I didn't hear the rest, so I asked about the phone

Chapter 6: The Skilled Nursing Facility

conversation. I was told that special authorization from the corporate pharmacy was needed to administer morphine to Mary Regina and she had already missed two scheduled doses.

Mary Regina seemed to suffer alternately with going to physical therapy without sufficient pain medication, being left in a wheelchair in the hallway in a stupor with her head dangling on her shoulder, or lying in bed "zonked" with drugs. I told any staffer who would listen that my mother had a sharp mind, and was suffering from the influence of medication. One nurse seemed to take an interest in getting the medication level correct. I suggested that the administration of pain medication be timed so that it was active in her system at the time of physical therapy. I said that at other times, Mary Regina did not need or want it.

Upon entering the hallway outside my mother's room early one morning, I overheard one particular nurse discussing Mary Regina's medication dosage with another staffer, and I was reassured by, and appreciative of, the nurse's interest. However, after Mary Regina's room was changed, that nurse was no longer her nurse.

One day early in Mary Regina's stay at MRNH, I asked to meet with a facility representative and presented a list of concerns.

During the meeting, I read out loud virtually word-for-word all 10 of the concerns I had written in my notebook in preparation for the meeting.

They were:

1. "No orientation. Limited orientation/form signing session held on 8 July about 4 p.m. Admission was 6 July about 2 p.m.

Chapter 6: The Skilled Nursing Facility

2. "Doctor care. In response to a question, I was told law only requires doctor visit to facility once per month. On initial visit, doctor made fast and loose decisions on pain medication changes. . . .
3. "Medication. (A) Upon walking past nurses' station, I heard staff member refer to "the problem with Regina Beerman." In response to my question, I was told she had missed two doses of pain medication because they needed narcotics authorization from their out-of-state corporate pharmacy. She had been undergoing painful therapy without adequate medication. (B) Over-medication. Apparently doctor's new pain medication puts her into a near stupor, quasi-unconscious in chair. How can she rehabilitate?
4. "Food. First night hot dog and beans. Second day lunch, chicken sandwich. Did not eat. Second day dinner, steak sandwich soaked in a plate of water, with bun actually dissolving. Did not eat. Did not eat at least first four meals. No one informed her she could get alternatives, as noted in (1) above – No orientation.
5. "Bells (chimes) ring incessantly. Apparently very slow response to calls.
6. "Bathroom cleanliness. After noticing urine smell in room on day 2, went in bathroom and was shocked to see unflushed toilet and soiled garment on floor. Told nurse, who cleaned up. Second room bathroom smells of urine and does not look clean.
7. "Treatment. On her first night, staff member got verbally aggressive when mom told staff member breathing treatment being given was discontinued by doctor at Mercy Hospital.
8. "Although mom unable to get out of bed on her own, staff not offering to help with bathroom.

Chapter 6: The Skilled Nursing Facility

9. "Apparent inadequate attention to personal appearance. Hair not brushed. Finally, on 8 July mom was helped to get dressed.
10. "Not assisting with eating and drinking. Note item 4. Can lead to malnutrition and dehydration."

I told a facility representative that the book, *Eldercare for Dummies*, said neglect is the most common form of abuse in nursing facilities, and as an example of neglect, the book listed "Not assisting with eating and drinking." I pointed out that the book noted that lack of assistance with eating and drinking can lead to malnutrition and dehydration. This proved to be prophetic in Mary Regina's case.

(The book also lists as indicators of neglect: "Ignoring call lights, buzzers, and cries for help.")

The representative told me that she would look into the medication problem and also put Mary Regina on a supplemental diet.

But the worst was yet to come.

I tried to manage my conduct and tactfully cajole the staff into taking care of my mother's needs. I did not want them to decide that I was a nuisance. Although things have changed since then, I was also vaguely aware that if the nursing home decided Mary Regina was not making progress with her therapy, and reported that to Medicare, Medicare might stop making payments. Or, I worried, maybe MRNH could simply kick my mother out, saying they did not think they could help her any further. I lacked essential knowledge about the system at this point, and once, feeling stressed, I picked an eldercare attorney out of

Chapter 6: The Skilled Nursing Facility

the yellow pages and called him to ask basic advice. While I was writing this book, I learned about the sources of help available to nursing home consumers. This is discussed in Chapter 15.

When the therapists came to pick up Mary Regina to take her to therapy in the downstairs therapy area, Mary Regina sometimes would tell them she did not want to go. Sometimes she would tell them "I can't." I would help them persuade her to go.

I felt that I shared some motivation with the therapy staff to get Mary Regina to therapy. I wanted Mary Regina to make progress and recover, and for Medicare to keep paying, and MRNH presumably wanted the income from Mary Regina's therapy sessions. I also believed that the therapists, unlike some other nursing home staff, truly wanted to help.

Meanwhile, I resolved to try to get my mother into the nearby four-star Golden Living facility.

I visited Golden Living and was impressed with the bright, cheery atmosphere. Both the staff and patients seemed to be happy.

One significant difference about Golden Living was that they gave each patient and prospective patients' families a list of all 24 core staff members, with first and last names, and titles, from the executive director to the central supply clerk. The personnel did not seem to mind being identified to the patients and their families.

The list was entitled, "Meet our team..." and the introduction stated: "These individuals work together as a team to design and carry out your interdisciplinary plan of care."

Chapter 6: The Skilled Nursing Facility

I found it interesting that MRNH did not seem eager to disclose to patients who was who on the MRNH staff. I was unaware of any list of MRNH staffers being provided to residents or their families.

I knew of only two physicians associated with MRNH. But Golden Living Center provided residents and their families with a list of 16 "attending physicians" complete with their phone numbers.

Further, Golden Living Center gave patients and prospective patients a list of 10 phone numbers of oversight entities ranging from their Corporate Hotline to the Governor's Action Line, the Medical Assistance Fraud Control Unit, and some patient advocate agencies, including the Area Ombudsman's name, address, and phone number. In contrast, I was not aware of the existence of any such entity as an ombudsman during Mary Regina's stay at MRNH. I did not read all of the Golden Living literature immediately or thoroughly. However, I perceived a significant difference between two-star MRNH and four-star Golden Living Center.

I took my cousin Ellen to tour Golden Living and we talked with patients and staff. Ellen and I decided to get Mary Regina transferred. I informed Mary Regina of my plan, while consoling her that she would not have to remain at MRNH much longer.

Mary Regina was in favor of changing nursing homes. "Get me out of here," she said. Unfortunately, I would have to share bad news with her later when I found I could not get her out.

On July 11, I informed MRNH that I planned to transfer my mother.

Chapter 6: The Skilled Nursing Facility

Then, one of those fateful events occurred that helped seal Mary Regina's doom. When Golden Living called MRNH on July 12 to arrange the transfer, they learned that Mary Regina had been diagnosed that very day through lab results with a contagious infection called Clostridium difficile, which causes uncontrollable diarrhea. Regulations required patients with "C-diff" to be isolated in a private room.

Golden Living told me they did not have an isolation room available, and put Mary Regina on a waiting list. After a number of daily calls to Golden Living about whether a vacancy had opened up, I concluded that Mary Regina probably was trapped in MRNH. I felt it was unlikely that a nursing home would accept transfer of a patient with C-diff. I was told that C-diff can last a long time.

According to a MRNH billing statement, the Medicare daily rate for a double-occupancy room was $304 per person, and the rate for an isolation room was only $330, so it appeared that if a nursing home used a potential double-occupancy room as an isolation room, it would be losing $278 per day ($304 X 2 persons = $608, minus $330 (the rate for an isolation room) = $278). Nevertheless, I called other nursing homes such as Little Sisters of the Poor and Vincentian, and actually visited and/or applied to some, but they said they had waiting lists.

Several emotionally troubling incidents happened to Mary Regina at MRNH. In one case, she had been taken, despite her reluctance, downstairs to physical therapy, where she was being helped to walk between two grab bars. There were about a half dozen other patients in the room working with therapists, and Mary Regina had an episode of diarrhea caused by the C-diff and had to be taken off the

Chapter 6: The Skilled Nursing Facility

floor to a bathroom to be cleaned up. This certainly was extremely humiliating for her.

On another occasion, while therapists were gently encouraging her to take steps, she lashed out at me, demanding to know, "How can you allow them to do this to your mother?" I noticed that the other people in the room -- patients, relatives, and staff -- turned to see what was going on. I couldn't tell if their faces reflected sympathy or disdain. I said to my mother, "Do you want to spend the rest of your life in a bed? That's what will happen if you don't do this." I was concerned that the hip must heal properly and that Mary Regina must re-acquire the ability to walk. The thought that her life was in danger did not enter my mind. My cousin Ellen witnessed this incident and later said some sympathetic words to me.

Believing that my brother-in-law had more influence with my mother than I did, I apprised him of the situation and asked him to talk with Mary Regina about doing her therapy. He did so by phone, and shortly thereafter even traveled from Michigan to visit her.

In private, I told Mary Regina that if she did not make progress with her therapy, or refused it, Medicare might stop paying. Later I would have doubts about whether I should have said this. But Mary Regina was quite rational when not zonked with drugs and it seemed to me at the time to be an appropriate topic for discussion.

I expected she would see the logic just as I did. And there had already been a serious consequence from Mary Regina's refusing treatment -- the blood transfusion at Mercy Hospital. Later, staff told me Mary Regina said she wanted to die. They quoted her as saying, "Just put me in a pine box." I wondered if this was a delayed sarcastic

Chapter 6: The Skilled Nursing Facility

response to my expression of concern about Medicare stopping payments.

On a third occasion, Mary Regina became very upset when staff came to get her for a shower. She was wheeled off under protest. When she came back she asked harshly of me, "How would you like to get stripped and dragged into a shower?" This gave me the mental image of her being dragged into a shower in a cold room with staff members pulling on both arms, although I really did not know what had happened.

In a separate, bizarre, experience that I went through with -- and in a sense, without -- my mother, we were both taken by ambulance on July 25 to the office of her hip surgeon so he could do a follow-up check of her hip-surgery site. Mary Regina, in my layman's estimation, was utterly unconscious for the trip and I do not think she even knew she had left MRNH. The surgeon's office was in South Side, Pittsburgh, about 12 miles from MRNH.

The ambulance could get no closer than a block away from the doctor's office to park. So Mary Regina was wheeled unconscious, with her mouth open, down South Side city sidewalks on a gurney, as I walked alongside. She was then taken into a building and up via an elevator into the doctor's waiting room, which was full of people waiting in chairs – the typical waiting room scene. Some of those waiting seemed horrified at the sight of Mary Regina, and perhaps they were getting premonitions of the fate they might encounter themselves someday. She looked like a corpse. The staff was at lunch, but after one staff member became aware of the presence of Mary Regina, they moved her out of sight back to an exam room right away.

Chapter 6: The Skilled Nursing Facility

A doctor commented that he was surprised at Mary Regina's condition because she had been alert the previous time he had seen her. Years later, I wondered whether Mary Regina should have been sent from the doctor's office to Mercy Hospital, right across the Birmingham Bridge from South Side, instead of being sent back to MRNH. I also wondered why I had not thought to suggest it to the doctors, and why someone at the doctor's office didn't think to do it.

After Mary Regina's death, I wrote a somewhat detailed outline of Mary Regina's experience at MRNH in a complaint to the Pennsylvania Department of Health. This is covered in Chapter 9.

In general, I thought that during her 21 days at MRNH, Mary Regina went through hell.

In my view, during this time, she was over- and under-medicated, contracted two different infections (C-Diff and a urinary tract infection); contracted pneumonia, which also could be considered an infection; suffered critical-level digoxin poisoning; had treatment by a psychiatrist delayed after she expressed a wish to die, possibly because of the digoxin poisoning; was neglected while dehydrated; began having blood in her stool; and was allowed to lose weight drastically while missing numerous meals.

Measured on June 30, 2011 at Mercy Hospital, her weight was 53.0 kg, or 116.85 pounds. After she was transferred to MRNH on July 6, the last weight I found written into MRNH records, on July 21, was 102.8 pounds. The Forbes Regional Hospital emergency room recorded her weight at 45.2 kg, or 99.65 pounds, on July 27 at 6 p.m. Mary Regina's admission benchmark weight at MRNH was

Chapter 6: The Skilled Nursing Facility

blank on an intake form that MRNH provided to me with the rest of her records after her death.

Mary Regina had been living alone independently before breaking her hip and going to MRNH for therapy after hip repair surgery at Mercy Hospital. She was described at Mercy Hospital as "pleasant" with an "optimistic prognosis."

In a report sent with Mary Regina to her hip surgeon on July 25, 2011, Mary Regina's therapist at MRNH wrote: "Unable to arouse for therapy 2() meds....Pt [Patient] is heavily medicated and has no desire to live or get better .... Pt did well at first but has gone downhill since."

A nurse told me on July 20 that Mary Regina looked dry. Although intravenous hydration treatment was ordered by a physician on July 23, MRNH allowed Mary Regina to languish without accomplishing the IV treatment until she was sent to the emergency room on July 27 for "dehydration" and decreased consciousness. After a complaint by me and an on-site survey, including a records review and interviews, the Pennsylvania Department of Health, Division of Nursing Care Facilities, cited MRNH for violating state and federal regulations regarding failure to implement the physician's order for an IV for Mary Regina. This is covered in Chapter 9.

I felt that certain quantifiable indicators were illustrative of the level of care provided to Mary Regina. One was the numerical change in her weight, and another was the number of days, or nursing shifts, that elapsed from the time Mary Regina was observed to be looking dry on July 20 until she was sent to the emergency room on July 27 for dehydration, without her ever effectively receiving the IV treatment ordered by the doctor on July 23. The

Chapter 6: The Skilled Nursing Facility

interval from July 20-27 could have encompassed as many as 21 nursing/staffing shifts. Another quantifiable factor was how many meals she had missed. I believe she missed, for example, about 15 consecutive meals over her last 5 days at MRNH, and others before that.

A MRNH report said staff inserted an IV line on July 23 but it infiltrated and was removed after a few hours. It was never reinserted. On its internet page, MRNH Health Services said "our professional staff provides comprehensive health care around the clock in a safe and comfortable environment." Under the heading, "Our Experience," the web page listed 15 points of medical services such as "Trach care," and "Stroke and neurological care." Prominently presented as the first item in the list of points under "our experience" was a bullet for "I.V. therapy."

Within 2 hours of her arrival at Forbes Regional Hospital from MRNH on July 27, Mary Regina was found to be suffering from a "critical" level of digoxin poisoning, a condition that I believe MRNH should have caught, because staff had promised me a review of her medications at a meeting on July 20. Such poisoning could account for many of the symptoms exhibited by Mary Regina while she was at MRNH, where she was given digoxin daily.

According to the *New York Times* Health Guide on March 21, 2016, digitalis (also known as digoxin) toxicity can result in confusion, irregular pulse, loss of appetite, nausea, vomiting, diarrhea, decreased consciousness, and difficulty breathing when lying down. The EMTs said Mary Regina had difficulty breathing while, presumably lying down, in the ambulance on the way to the emergency room on July 27.

Chapter 6: The Skilled Nursing Facility

Some medical guidelines call for monitoring of digoxin levels in patients, especially when a patient is also on Lipitor. MRNH was giving Mary Regina a generic equivalent of Lipitor each day.

MRNH told Mary Regina's family that MRNH was legally required to have patients seen by a doctor only once per month, and that Mary Regina's former regular doctor for over 20 years had "no authority" at MRNH. To my knowledge, normally no physician was on the premises, and nurses would phone a physician and request orders. The physician would later call back with orders and occasionally physicians would come in.

After MRNH told the family that Mary Regina had exhibited psychiatric problems and said she wanted to die ("Just put me in a pine box"), staff told the family on July 20 that the psychiatrist was not due in until the 26th, but they would have a regular doctor prescribe an antidepressant in the meantime. I suppressed my reaction, and did not insist on an immediate examination by a psychiatrist, because I was afraid Mary Regina would be transferred to a facility for mental patients. In retrospect, this fear almost certainly was unfounded. My record for sound decision making was not good during these times.

The staff repeatedly gave Mary Regina doses of morphine and/or Klonopin. According to Wikipedia, Klonopin is a medication used to prevent and treat seizures and panic disorder, and for the movement disorder known as akathisia. It is a tranquilizer of the benzodiazepine class. It begins having an effect within an hour and lasts between 6 and 12 hours. Common side effects include sleepiness, poor coordination, and agitation. It may increase risk of suicide.

Chapter 6: The Skilled Nursing Facility

Mary Regina, in my layman's view, was left to lie unconscious from drugs around the clock on some days, and for stretches of multiple days, and she was unable to eat or drink, even though I believed she had not complained of pain or exhibited signs of anxiety.

I visited the nursing home at 5:30 the morning of July 26, 2011, confirmed what I considered to be improper drugging, and complained in writing. MRNH's director of nursing called me on July 29, subsequent to an internal inquiry, to tell me that there was "no reason she [MRNH staff member] should have administered the medication. [She] should have notified her supervisor. We are addressing that with [the staff member]."

Later, I found out that a person with the same name as the MRNH staff person at issue in my written complaint was registered with the state as a nurse's aide. I subsequently confirmed with the Pennsylvania Department of Health that nurse's aides were not allowed to give medication in a nursing home setting in Pennsylvania.

Responding to my request for Mary Regina's records, MRNH sent a collection of records, including at least one that had been altered. This collection of records was missing records pertaining to promised investigations of rough treatment of Mary Regina and of failure by MRNH to deliver food trays to her for an entire day after she had been moved from one room to another, and family complaints about inappropriate drugging. Also missing were documents that MRNH had coaxed Mary Regina into signing while she was drugged.

I believed the treatment of, or neglect of, Mary Regina ultimately proved fatal, when she died at Forbes Regional

Chapter 6: The Skilled Nursing Facility

Hospital officially of sepsis, pneumonia due to a bedridden state, and other complications on August 7, 2011.

***

As it became evident that Mary Regina's rehabilitation therapy might not succeed, I inquired what would happen to Mary Regina if her Medicare payments stopped, since I could not seem to get her transferred to another facility.

A MRNH administrator said that she would be permitted to remain at MRNH if she were approved for Medicaid or if the family paid the cost. During Mary Regina's stay at MRNH, I filled out the Medical Assistance (Medicaid) Financial Assistance Eligibility Application for Long-Term Care, Support, and Services provided to me by the nursing home. This required much effort, such as gathering many pages of supporting documentation and a visit to the Allegheny County Department of Public Welfare (DPW) office in downtown Pittsburgh, while I was in a state of stress and varying levels of mental fog.

The documentation provided by me included power of attorney papers, an affidavit from the manager of Mary Regina's apartment building stating how many years and months she had been at the residence, her rent amount, a general summary fact sheet, birth certificate, Pennsylvania driver's license, Social Security card, health insurance cards and certificates of insurance, multiple monthly statements of income and bank statements, proof of a burial agreement, and names, addresses, and phone numbers of life insurance companies and insurance policy statements.

I had been advised that since most families would quickly be wiped out financially by the cost of nursing home care, it was wise to apply for Medicaid before, rather

Chapter 6: The Skilled Nursing Facility

than after, the family's assets had been depleted. Medicaid eligibility was based on the patient's and the patient's spouse's assets, not the children's, so the children were not required to spend down their own assets to qualify a patient for Medicaid.

On August 11, 2011, several days after Mary Regina's death, I received a letter from the Pennsylvania Department of Public Welfare informing me that Mary Regina was not eligible for Medicaid benefits based on her income of $1,356 per month, which was $150 over the limit of $1,226 at that time.

This made me wonder where the estimated $9,000 per month, or roughly $300 per day of semi-private room cost of a nursing home would have come from after the 100 days covered by Medicare for rehabilitative care ended. I wondered whether the denial could have been appealed and the math recomputed to show negative monthly net income after nursing home fees if a nursing home became Mary Regina's permanent residence. Because of her death, I never had to pursue that issue.

While researching this book, I attempted to contact the DPW to ask whether Mary Regina would have become eligible for Medicaid when Medicare stopped payments after 100 days, and Mary Regina was faced with $9,000 a month in nursing home bills. I became exasperated after a half dozen unsuccessful calls including one in which one DPW employee responded to my question with the remark, "I have no idea."

I finally was told by a person at the Allegheny County Area Agency on Aging that it was likely Mary Regina would have been able to have Medicaid pay for her nursing home had she lived.

Chapter 6: The Skilled Nursing Facility

I had only about 10 months of nursing home room-and-board costs in my savings, and I also had my wife and children to think about with regard to financial management.

Had Mary Regina been able to move to an assisted living facility after her rehabilitation, the cost would have been about one third of the cost of a nursing home. However, generally speaking, there is no government subsidy such as Medicaid available to pay for assisted living facilities, except for war-time veterans and their spouses, who may be able to get an Aid and Attendance Benefit.

It was some comfort to me that my brother-in-law generously offered to split the cost of an assisted living facility with me, and he also attempted to get Mary Regina transferred to a nice nursing home in Michigan, where he lived. I considered renting a motorhome for Mary Regina's trip from Pittsburgh to Michigan. While Mary Regina was at Forbes Regional Hospital, her doctor said that she would not be ready to be moved out of state for a few weeks. However, she died before becoming stable enough to make the move.

Mary Regina's charges to Medicare from MRNH amounted to $11,404 for 21 days. These included $1,410 for physical therapy, $1,920 for occupational therapy, and $6,777 for room and board, with 15 days at $330 per day for the isolation room, and 6 days at $304 for a semiprivate room. Later, Medicare was billed another $10,220 for hospital bills after MRNH sent Mary Regina to Forbes Regional Hospital for treatment of various conditions, including some she acquired while at MRNH. There also were charges to Mary Regina's AARP supplemental

Chapter 6: The Skilled Nursing Facility

medical insurance, which, incidentally, she always had been pleased with.

It occurred to me years later that Mary Regina might not have needed a nursing home, if not for the conditions she acquired while in a nursing home. I wondered whether we would have been better off if I had taken Mary Regina home to her apartment from the hospital, and spent the 21 days I had spent at the nursing home staying instead with her at her apartment as she recovered. Maybe we could have had therapists come to the apartment, and I could have extended my stay in Pittsburgh if necessary. Maybe that was not a realistic option, or maybe it was, but it simply did not occur to me at the time.

On April 7, 2016, the following complaint about a nursing home was displayed on a website. It had been posted in August 2013, about 2 years after Mary Regina's death on August 7, 2011. It reinforced my belief that Mary Regina's experience was not unique.

"My father spent several months at this facility and I would NOT recommend it. The care was mediocre at best-- they had a few good nurses and therapists who have since left, but most of the staff was lazy.

"My father was bed-bound and completely dependent on them for his care. He had COPD and CHF [congestive heart failure] (along with getting pneumonia frequently) and had a very difficult time breathing. **He would often have to wait for close to an hour to get a response if he rang for help** *and then if he got upset and made smart comments, they seemed to be out to get him and responded like adolescents who were "getting even" with someone they didn't like. I am not saying that my father should have been rude to them, however, we had the "good" staff*

Chapter 6: The Skilled Nursing Facility

members even tell us that he was usually justified in his complaints and they never had any problem with him (because those few did their jobs and were not just trying to get out of work).

"One time when we did complain about something that happened, the way they "dealt" with it was to ask the staff member involved, who of course denied it, so it was immediately let go.

"After my dad was taken to the hospital for the last time, we received a phone call and written notification that under Medicaid guidelines, they would hold his room for so many days, and then we would have the option of paying out-of-pocket if we wanted it held longer. My mother went in the day after she received the letter to pack my dad's things and was stopped by a nurse midway down the hall saying that his room had already been filled (while they were supposed to still be holding it) and that the nurse had packed his belongings and put them in storage a couple days prior. When my mom got his two boxes home, everything (including all of his clothes that had been neatly hung in his closet) were literally just thrown in a heap in the boxes out of spite.

"When I called to inquire about why they had filled his room when they were still supposed to be holding it, I was told that the administrator would call me back, which of course never happened. In addition, we also could have reported them to the Health Department on more than one occasion because my dad's nasal cannula would fall onto the filthy floor and the nurses would just pick it up and put it right back into his nose--without changing it, cleaning it, or anything. No wonder he got MRSA [a virulent staff infection] and a multitude of other infections!

Chapter 6: The Skilled Nursing Facility

"If you care about your loved one, DON'T send them to [this nursing home]!"

Chapter 7: Western Pennsylvania Hospital; Forbes Regional Campus

I flew home to New Mexico for a respite on July 27. I had been spending a lot of time sitting at Mary Regina's bedside while she didn't even know I was there. I missed my wife, and when I would see other people with their dogs I would miss my dog, too.

I had been trying to get home and had rearranged my flight and rental car plans several times over almost a month in Pittsburgh as Mary Regina's condition changed. Flight and rental car reservations had to be made at least several days in advance or the price would be exorbitant. I used Southwest Airlines because if I canceled, Southwest would allow me to bank the cost of the ticket with Southwest for future use, so I wouldn't lose my money altogether as with other airlines. But the price of a short-lead-time flight would nevertheless be very expensive.

When I got off the plane in El Paso on the way home to Las Cruces I had a phone message from the nursing home telling me my mother had been taken to a hospital.

Chapter 7: Forbes Hospital

When I called Forbes Regional Hospital, I found they had quickly diagnosed Mary Regina's problems and had some initial success in bringing her back from critical condition. They had done a chest x-ray and a CT scan of her head, as well as lab tests. They inserted an IV line called a "PIC" line into her jugular vein to treat dehydration.

A Forbes intervention specialist told me on the phone that Mary Regina was suffering from digoxin poisoning and the specialist mentioned some digoxin blood level numbers that I did not understand. Later I saw the lab report, which stated: "This Report Requires an *Immediate* Phone Call to the Physician." It said, "DIGOXN 3.0. critical," and contained control notes for the date and time the physician was notified of the digoxin level, and the physician's name. This showed the serious nature of the poisoning.

Mary Regina was admitted into the telemetry unit for a urinary tract infection, a change in mental status, the toxic digitalis level, and electrocardiogram changes. I was impressed with how quickly Forbes had diagnosed Mary Regina's conditions and acted to rectify them.

The next day a doctor from Forbes told me my mother had been stabilized and it was not necessary for me to fly back to Pittsburgh immediately.

Mary Regina went through some relatively good days and bad ones at Forbes. I would call and talk briefly with Mary Regina, who sounded lethargic when I called, or, if she was not awake, I would talk with her nurse, who was very pleasant and willing to advise me of my mother's condition in detail. At one point, on July 31, Mary Regina was processed for release. However, my cousin, Ellen, and

Chapter 7: Forbes Hospital

I told Mary Regina's Forbes doctor that we did not want Mary Regina to be returned to MRNH, and the outplacement specialist at Forbes began making calls to four- and five-star nursing homes suggested by me.

A Forbes social worker spoke with me on August 2 about transfer and I asked that referrals be sent to Little Sisters of the Poor; Vincentian; Marian Manor; Golden Living Center; John J. Kane, Scott or Glen Hazel locations; or Baptist skilled nursing facilities. The social worker notified me on August 3 that Marian Manor had no beds available, but that she was still working on placement.

I would also talk regularly with Mary Regina's primary doctor at Forbes, Dr. Palaniapp Muthappan, who eventually suggested that because Mary Regina was encountering new complications as well as suffering from chronic ones, he could arrange for her to be placed at a "long-term acute care hospital." This type of hospital was a new concept to me, but as the doctor explained it, I thought it was a great idea and I was grateful for the doctor's suggestion.

Long-term acute care hospitals furnish medical and rehabilitative care to individuals with clinically complex problems, such as multiple acute or chronic conditions, who need hospital-level care for relatively extended periods. Chronic conditions could include prolonged ventilator use or weaning, intensive respiratory care, and multiple IV medications or transfusions.

Such facilities qualify for Medicare payment if they meet certain conditions, including Medicare's conditions of participation for acute care (regular) hospitals, and if they have an average inpatient length of stay greater than 25 days. Medicare recognized 436 long-term acute care

Chapter 7: Forbes Hospital

hospitals nationally in 2011, and such hospitals are still part of the system today.

This suggestion seemed to me, as a layman, to be a good match to Mary Regina's needs, considering her condition after her stay at MRNH.

I had acquired a strong appreciation of the difference between hospital care and nursing home care.

Forbes proved to be a source of information that documented Mary Regina's condition when she was admitted to Forbes, as well as her treatment during her time at Forbes. The records were neat, orderly, and generally computerized. The Forbes records even included a chart listing all of the medical personnel involved in the case, along with their initials, so that records could be matched to the person who created them. When I procured my mother's medical records, I received 373 pages of mostly computerized records from Forbes from my mother's 10 days there, for a fee of $192 from a record service company. I obtained about 125 pages covering 21 days from MRNH, for a fee of $182. I concluded that the purchase of the records was a good investment.

I believed that the records illustrated the vastly different levels of care between a skilled nursing home such as MRNH and a hospital. I noted, for example, that Forbes had done a psych evaluation on Mary Regina without even asking me. In contrast, MRNH had told me my mother needed one, but they put it off until the doctor's regular scheduled visit to the nursing home 6 days later. Mary Regina also received other treatments at Forbes such as a gastrointestinal procedure and evaluation conducted by a Forbes team because of internal bleeding.

Chapter 7: Forbes Hospital

I concluded that if you are more than slightly sick, you had better be in a hospital, not a nursing home.

I gained an insight into medical care provided to my mother by going through about 500 pages of hospital and nursing home records. This awareness caused me to change my mind about proposed legislation limiting people's right to sue in response to healthcare malpractice. I am now convinced that the right of patients to sue should be preserved. It is desirable for a facility to do everything it can for a patient, even if the motivation might be a fear of lawsuits. Conversely, a limitation on such lawsuits could result in some facilities cutting corners on costs and becoming lax on care. Laws and lawsuits are needed because some people won't do the right thing unless they are compelled to.

I thought that myself and others probably had unrealistic expectations regarding skilled nursing homes because of the words "skilled" and "nursing" in their names. It later was some comfort to me to know that at least in Mary Regina's final 10 days, at Forbes, she had gotten quality care, and Forbes probably did everything that could have been done for her.

On the day of her death, August 7, Mary Regina's Forbes doctor, Dr. Muthappan, wrote an addendum to the discharge summary stating that in the interim after he aborted her discharge on August 1, Mary Regina developed internal bleeding and a gastrointestinal evaluation was done. The evaluation identified a duodenal ulcer that could have been the cause of the bleeding. He said Mary Regina then developed pneumonia and acute respiratory failure. She continued to decline and the doctor requested "comfort measures" be taken.

Chapter 7: Forbes Hospital

I arrived from New Mexico the night of August 6 and Mary Regina died the morning of August 7. I had not known my mother was dying when I embarked on the flight to Pittsburgh. I had scheduled the trip some time earlier, and the doctor knew I was due in on the 6th.

Mary Regina was unconscious when I arrived after driving straight from the airport to the hospital. I slept in a chair in her room for some time and then noticed that she had stopped breathing.

I squeezed her arm and told her to rest in peace. But I was emotionally inert.

I felt differently than the way I had when my father died. He died suddenly at a relatively young age while he was enjoying himself somewhat during his retirement. For my father, I had strong feelings of grief and loss, but I did not permit them to overwhelm me. In the case of my mother, at the time of her death, she was much older; she was suffering; and her prospects for a good quality of life seemed very poor. Although I loved her to some degree, and she probably loved me, our relationship had never been warm, nor our bond strong.

Chapter 8:
A Funeral Home Hassle

After a Forbes Regional Hospital nurse confirmed that Mary Regina had died, the nurse asked who would handle the funeral arrangements, and whether the nurse should call anyone. I gave her the name of the funeral home where Mary Regina had a pre-paid plan. The nurse called the funeral home. That step went very smoothly. The funeral home acted quickly in picking up the body.

When I went to my mother's apartment building to inform the manager that Mary Regina had died, I was surprised when the manager, who was a Catholic nun, asked me if I had called a priest. I had to say no, and felt some embarrassment about telling that to a nun. Mary Regina had asked me to arrange for her to see a priest while she was at MRNH and I had done so. However, it did not occur to me that someone who had gone to Mass each morning during her later years would need a priest at her deathbed, especially if she was unconscious or had already died.

Chapter 8: A Funeral Home Hassle

I would be in for another surprise later when I called Mary Regina's designated funeral home to discuss the arrangements. The funeral director told me that my mother had no prepaid funeral plan. The funeral director was adamant. "Many elderly ladies look into getting a plan, but they never pay the money. They end up thinking they have a plan, but they don't," he said.

I knew that Mary Regina had a prepaid plan, and I told the funeral director that my mother had been quite in command of her faculties when she told me she had a plan. The funeral director refused to entertain the possibility. He told me I would have to produce a contract.

I was annoyed. I had some of my mother's papers in New Mexico, and some were in her apartment in Brookline. There were one or two folders with many pages about the prepaid funeral plan. I needed one particular page with the signature of the person who sold the plan. I had to call my wife to have her search the pertinent papers at home in New Mexico while I checked at my mother's apartment. Fortunately, we located the contract. "That's what I need," said the funeral director without embarrassment when I described the paper to him. "My secretary must have misfiled our copy," he said.

I resented that the funeral director had caused me an irritating inconvenience when he should have been facilitating things. I wondered what would have happened if I had not been able to find the specified piece of paper. Presumably I would have had to pay for the funeral a second time. How many sole-surviving sons living on the other side of the country possibly would be unaware that a prepaid plan existed, or would accept the funeral director's story about old women deluding themselves into thinking they have prepaid funeral plans when they don't?

Chapter 8: A Funeral Home Hassle

Later I would encounter another questionable situation when my mother's casket was being closed. Mary Regina wanted an urn with some of her daughter's ashes to be buried with her. My brother-in-law asked me to make sure the urn with his late wife's ashes was put into the casket. However, the funeral director told me that the law did not allow me to remain in the room when the casket lid was closed and locked. I did not argue but I thought this was a strange law. Because I could not be in the room when the casket was locked, I lacked certainty that the urn was actually locked into the casket.

Despite the existence of the prepaid funeral contract, which was based on prepaid insurance policies that covered the funeral, I was nevertheless billed $535 for the funeral. The funeral director said the charge was for items not covered by the prepaid contract.

Later, because one of Mary Regina's fellow residents of Creedmoor Court had mentioned that she was planning to buy a prepaid funeral, I made it a point to tell the manager of the apartment building, which was full of old ladies, what had happened. I asked the manager to warn the residents to make sure their prepaid funeral contracts were kept in a safe place where they would be accessible to their designated administrators or executors.

The Pennsylvania State Board of Funeral Directors provides an online search database of funeral director and supervisor licensees. A search for Mary Regina's funeral director showed that he had both a director's license and a supervisor's license. The database search function reported: "No disciplinary actions were found for this license." I did not check for complaints.

I did not search all of the Board's regulations, but a

Chapter 8: A Funeral Home Hassle

staffer at the Board office told me there was no law preventing a family member from being present when a casket was closed and locked.

At the funeral Mass, I delivered a eulogy, in which I focused on Mary Regina's independent nature:

"She had a hard life, in some respects. She certainly did not enjoy all of the comforts that money can buy. For about 50 of her 86 years, she encountered one devastating illness after another. Her last months were especially difficult.

"But she coped admirably, as long as she could. And she tried to maintain her independence. She even arranged her own funeral.

"Despite her problems, Regina was a wealthy woman in terms of spiritual, intangible possessions. She possessed a wonderful home in the Creedmoor Court community next door to this church, which is where she wanted to be .... She drew strength and comfort from her faith .... She possessed the love of many people .... She left a legacy of good memories in the hearts of friends and relatives .... and four grandchildren"

On the afternoon of the funeral and burial, I held a catered reception luncheon for about 40 people at Creedmoor Court. The building manager graciously allowed me to use the community room. It was a very pleasant setting, and it was convenient for those residents of Mary Regina's building who wanted to attend. Some residents brought, from their apartments upstairs, desserts to complement the catered meal. The room had a few memorial plaques on the wall commemorating former residents who had died. A plaque was mounted later in memory of Mary Regina.

PART THREE: Government Oversight of Nursing Homes

Managers knew when inspections were coming.
— Confidential witnesses

Chapter 9: The Pennsylvania Department Of Health; Inspectors Under Scrutiny

The Pennsylvania Department of Health (DOH), Division of Nursing Care Facilities (DNCF), Bureau of Facility Licensure and Certification, is responsible for licensing and overseeing Pennsylvania's nursing care facilities. In September 2016, there were about 700 nursing care facilities with 80,000 residents in Pennsylvania. The number of facilities had declined only slightly since 2012, the year DOH investigated my complaint, when there were 710.

Chapter 9: The Pennsylvania Department of Health

During my research for this book, the DOH came under indirect scrutiny from the Pennsylvania attorney general, as well as a Washington, DC private law firm known for suing nursing homes (Chapter 10), and under direct scrutiny from the Pennsylvania auditor general (Chapter 11) and journalists (this chapter).

In June 2012, according to the DOH website, the DOH was doing approximately 5,000 nursing home surveys (inspections) of all types per year. This would equate to a benchmark average of about seven surveys per year per facility, although some facilities were inspected more frequently and others less frequently, based on their past performance and numbers of complaints filed against them. Surveys included licensure and certification surveys, follow-up surveys, and complaint investigations.

In a 2016 report, the state auditor general said DOH did 7,235 surveys/inspections of all types during the 22 months from January 1, 2014 through October 31, 2015, for a rate of about 3,950 per year. In 2014-15, at 3,950 surveys per year, and about 700 facilities, the DOH was conducting surveys/inspections at an average rate of 5.6 per facility per year. The 5.6 number represents a decline of 20 percent from the seven per year in 2012.

In 2016, the DOH said it had a DNCF staffing level of 146. A workload of 3,950 surveys/inspections per year for 146 employees would equate to 27 surveys/inspections per employee per year, or 2.25 per employee per month. However, some inspections use multiple inspectors.

***

In late December 2011 or early January 2012, I submitted a two-page, single-spaced complaint to the

Chapter 9: The Pennsylvania Department of Health

Pennsylvania DOH, DNCF, Bureau of Facility Licensure and Certification, through its complaint website. My strongly worded complaint covered the issues raised in Chapter 6, and I won't repeat them here. But the complaint began: "This is a preliminary complaint to ensure my complaint gets on the record before [MRNH's] updated rating is issued in early 2012. I have documentation and would like to talk with an investigator."

When I called to find out whether DOH had received my complaint over the internet, as I hoped to talk with an investigator, I was surprised to learn the investigation had already been completed, with a 1-day onsite "abbreviated survey." The DOH completed a letter report giving me the results of the investigation within 2 days of its on-site abbreviated survey.

I was disappointed when I read the DOH response to the complaint. I felt that the DOH investigators had disregarded most of the issues I raised.

In the letter, which was dated January 25, 2012, the DOH described its investigation and the results. My thoughts about the process and the findings appear in bold italics within the letter, quoted here, as follows.

"Thank you for the correspondence regarding the care and services provided to your mother, Mary Regina Beerman, while a resident of [MRNH]. As a result, a surveyor visited the facility on January 23, 2012, to look into your concerns." (*I noted that my request to talk with an investigator and my offer to provide documentation had been ignored. If DOH had contacted me before visiting the nursing home or before issuing its letter report, I could have pointed out materially pertinent facts.*)

Chapter 9: The Pennsylvania Department of Health

"During our visit we reviewed clinical records and facility reports and interviewed staff. You expressed concern about your mother's weight loss. The clinical records indicated that the facility staff were aware of her poor appetite and that an appetite stimulant and supplements were ordered and later increased. There is documentation of refusal of meals. We were not able to determine that trays were not delivered to your mother."

(I felt this reply was both nonresponsive and misleading. I could have informed the investigator(s) that "refusals of meals" were actually documented consequences of Mary Regina lying virtually unconscious for days.

MRNH was "aware" of my mother's nutrition problem because I complained to them about it. The issue was not whether they were aware of the problem, but rather that they did not deal effectively with it.

The reply did not specifically state the scope of the review -- what was reviewed? DOH ignored my complaint about poor response time to call chimes. There was no mention of staffing adequacy in the DOH letter. Staffing was key to providing the care necessary and for avoiding problems arising from neglect. Did the records show there was an authorized nurse on duty at the time a nurse's aide allegedly gave medication to my mother without authorization? Most comments about survey findings were general in nature and neither quantified nor date-specific. The report simply stated DOH was "unable to determine" information that I thought they should have been able to determine from the records. Facts were missing, such as Mary Regina's weight at admission and discharge and the number and dates of all instances of "refusal of meals.")

"You also expressed concern that your mother developed bedsores. Measures to prevent skin breakdown were ordered for your mother on admission and were documented as provided. Skin assessments were completed at intervals and did not indicate skin breakdown." *(MRNH's own records show MRNH notified my cousin that Mary Regina had an abrasion on her elbow. Hospital admission records also documented that skin problems existed when Mary Regina arrived at the hospital from MRNH.)*

Chapter 9: The Pennsylvania Department of Health

"The clinical record indicated your mother did develop C-diff while at the facility. Review of current infections at the time of your mother's stay did not indicate any pattern of occurrence of C-diff at the facility." *(I did not believe the important issue was that there was no pattern of C-diff. I believed the relevant point was that my mother contracted multiple infections at MRNH. The letter mentioned neither her urinary tract infection nor pneumonia (an apparent infection, for which Mary Regina was treated with an antibiotic and oxygen.)*

"The clinical record indicated that pain medication was ordered on admission and changed shortly thereafter to a more effective one. The record also indicated that the dosage of pain medication was adjusted in response to your mother's condition. There was not an indication that a medication was not available from the pharmacy. Medications, including Digoxin, were administered in accordance with doctor's orders."

(The pain medication dosage was changed as a result of my complaints, which were documented in the records, not in a response by MRNH to my 'mother's condition,' as stated in the DOH letter. On what basis did the inspector conclude that medication was changed to "a more effective one"? Did the inspector mean more effective at putting my mother into a stupor or rendering her unconscious for days? A pain assessment in Mary Regina's records showed she told MRNH her pain level ranged from zero to three on a 10-point scale. On the other hand, I believed the fact that Mary Regina missed two consecutive doses of medication (possibly covering 16 hours) while MRNH attempted to get authorization from its corporate pharmacy should have been evident in the nursing records. The time- and date-stamped faxes requesting and providing the corporate authorization for morphine should have been in the records. I felt the choice of language, "There was not an indication," was obfuscating, vague, and ambiguous. Staff should have been asked to affirm or deny the complaint.

Furthermore, I felt that the claim that medications were "administered in accordance with doctor's orders" was no excuse for allowing Mary Regina to lie unconscious for days or for her suffering from critical digoxin poisoning, as was documented upon her arrival at the hospital emergency room. I wondered, aren't

Chapter 9: The Pennsylvania Department of Health

nurses supposed to monitor the effects of medications they give? Also, I believed the doctor had ordered that pain medication be given as needed, or as requested, yet there was an indication medication was given when not requested or needed. The response also did not address MRNH's internal inquiry into my written complaint about excessive medication and possible administration of medication by a nurse's aide who was not authorized to do so. This was precisely a case of medication NOT being administered in accordance with doctor's orders. I reasoned that if Mary Regina was being rendered unconscious ("zonked") and unable to eat or drink by drugging, this was likely the root cause of the dehydration and other problems.

Finally, the letter did not mention that a nursing note from July 26 at 4:45 p.m., the day before Mary Reginia was sent to the emergency room, stated a nurse spoke to a doctor "regarding morphine zonking.")

"The physician notes indicate that your mother was seen several times while in the facility and laboratory studies were ordered by the physician based on those examinations."

(This statement was vague and misleading. I believed it was irrelevant that my mother was seen "several times." She had not been seen enough. The investigation should have documented times and dates when a physician saw Mary Regina. MRNH's practice was to phone a doctor and get orders from the doctor by phone.

The actual citation ultimately issued by the Health Department said: "The meal consumption report indicated that Resident R1 refused meals on 7/23, 7/24, and 7/25/11, and listed amount consumed as 0% eaten." I believed this in effect documented that Mary Regina had lain unconscious for at least those 3 days, missing nine meals on those days alone, and she probably also did not eat at all on July 26 or July 27, when she was sent to the emergency room, and on other days. If she was seen by a physician during the days she was languishing without the IV that a doctor had ordered on July 23, why didn't the doctor do something? The citation eventually issued said, "During an interview on 1/23/11, at 1:20 p.m., Registered Nurse (RN) Employee E1 acknowledged that there was no indication that the physician was made aware when resident R1 refused meals on 7/23, 7/24, and 7/25/11." Also, MRNH delayed having Mary Regina seen by a

Chapter 9: The Pennsylvania Department of Health

psychiatrist for multiple days, until his or her regularly scheduled visit.)

"Your mother's clinical records indicated that following receipt of laboratory reports, intravenous fluids were ordered by the physician. A concern was identified with the facility's process for implementation of those orders and communication with the physician regarding them. The facility will be required to submit a corrective action plan." (*The euphemism, "A concern was identified," glossed over the fact that this situation actually involved a "violation" of state and federal regulations, not to mention that the violation resulted in Mary Regina's being sent to the emergency room at a hospital where she died 10 days later. I might never have known about the violation if I had not checked.)*

"This facility has been surveyed several times during the past year. All prior reports can be viewed at the facility or on the Pennsylvania Department of Health website." (*I had to look up the records for prior surveys to find out the results. The citation DOH eventually issued showed previous citations of MRNH on March 25, June 20, and December 21, 2011 for violating Pennsylvania Code sections requiring that residents receive treatments as prescribed.*)

I found myself wondering whether any citation would have been issued if I had not complained so strongly about the letter. The letter did not mention any "citation," or "violation." It said only that a "concern was identified" and that a corrective action plan would be required.

When I complained to the DOH Pittsburgh office supervisor about the DOH response to my complaint, I did not have the benefit of knowing information contained in the actual citation that was eventually issued. I had to wait to see the actual citation for the failure to provide the intravenous fluids because the DOH allowed the nursing home a period of advance notice to respond before releasing the citation to the complainant.

Chapter 9: The Pennsylvania Department of Health

The DOH eventually cited MRNH only for one instance of noncompliance with Title 42, Code of Federal Regulations (CFR), and Title 28, Pennsylvania Code.

The citation statement of deficiencies said:

"Based on an Abbreviated Survey in response to a complaint completed on January 24, 2012, it was determined that [MRNH] was not in compliance with the following requirements of 42 CFR Part 483, Subpart B, Requirements for Long-Term Facilities and the 28 Pa. Code, Commonwealth of Pennsylvania Long-Term Care Licensure Regulations.

"483.25(j) SUFFICIENT FLUID TO MAINTAIN HYDRATION

"The facility must provide each resident with sufficient fluid intake to maintain proper hydration and health.

"This REQUIREMENT was not met as evidenced by:

"Based on clinical record review and staff interview, it was determined that the facility failed to maintain hydration for one of seven residents (Resident R1).

"Findings include:

"The admitting record indicated that Resident R1 was admitted on 7/6/11, following repair of fractured hip, with diagnoses that included high blood pressure, chronic obstructive pulmonary disease (COPD), atrial fibrillation (irregular heart rhythm) and anxiety.

"The nutritional progress notes dated 7/21/11, indicated intakes were poor at around 38% for 20 meals and "nurses state IV fluids are being considered."

Chapter 9: The Pennsylvania Department of Health

(As of July 21, Mary Regina actually had been at MRNH for 15 days, so I thought 45 meals (three per day) should have been accounted for. The process used to arrive at the 38-percent figure was not disclosed. Also, there were numerous instances of zero meal consumption after July 21.)

"Resident R1's laboratory report dated 7/23/11, indicated an elevated BUN (blood urea nitrogen test to determine kidney function).

"Nurse's notes dated 7/23/11, indicated that the physician was aware of Resident R1's laboratory report and ordered intravenous fluids (IV through the veins) to be administered.

"Nurse's notes dated 7/23/11, at 9:45 p.m., indicated that an IV was inserted in Resident's arm.

"Nurse's notes dated 7/24/11, at 3:00 a.m., indicated that Resident R1's IV infiltrated (fluid leaking into the tissue surrounding the veins) and the line was pulled. The clinical record did not indicate that an attempt was made to restart Resident R1's IV or that the physician was made aware that the IV line was pulled.

"The meal consumption report indicated that Resident R1 refused meals on 7/23, 7/24, and 7/25/11, and listed amount consumed as 0% eaten. The clinical record did not indicate the physician was made aware of Resident R1's refusal of meals for three days.

"Nurse's notes dated 7/26/11, at 4:45 p.m., indicated the physician was made aware that Resident R1 had no IV access.

"The physician discharge summary indicated that Resident R1 became very weak, was not eating, had poor IV access, became dehydrated and was transferred to the hospital. [*Actually, MRNH did not send Mary Regina to the*

Chapter 9: The Pennsylvania Department of Health

hospital emergency room until late afternoon, July 27, about 24 hours after the July 26, 4:45 p.m. nurse's note cited above. I also thought the citation understated the seriousness of Mary Regina's condition when she was sent to the hospital by calling her "very weak."]

"During an interview on 1/23/12, at 1:20 p.m., Registered Nurse (RN) Employee E1 acknowledged that there was no indication that the physician was made aware when Resident R1 refused meals on 7/23, 7/24, and 7/25/11. RN Employee E1 also confirmed there was no indication that an attempt was made to restart Resident R1's IV or that the physician was notified of the lack of IV access until 7/26/11.

"28 Pa Code: 211.10(c) Resident care policies. Previously cited 3/35(sic)/11.

"28 Pa. Code 211.12(d)(1)(5) Nursing services. Previously cited 12/21/11, 6/20/11, 3/25/11."

Adding insult to injury, the citation had a code in the margin: "SS=D." I found out in February 2016 that this cryptic code indicates Scope and Severity equals D. About 4 years after the code was assigned, I found out that the code D means "No Actual Harm with Potential for More than Minimal Harm that is Not Immediate Jeopardy," or in short, "**No Actual Harm**," even though DOH personnel knew my mother had died.

During my call to the DOH Pittsburgh Office to complain about the investigation results in 2012, I was told that investigators were allowed to consider only information provided to them by the nursing home during the 1-day investigatory visit there – not information provided by me subsequent to my complaint. The DOH refused to consider documents that I had, such as hospital

Chapter 9: The Pennsylvania Department of Health

records citing "poisoning occurring at/in a residential institution," or even copies of nursing home records that I had but which the Health Department investigators apparently had not seen.

Further, they refused to return to the facility to talk to the director of nursing, who had not been there on the day of their "abbreviated survey" visit. As noted earlier, the nursing home director of nursing told me in response to an internal MRNH complaint I filed that a MRNH staff member who had given Mary Regina medication should not have done so, and should have consulted a supervisor. However, the DOH stuck to its position that there was no medication error found at MRNH.

Later, in 2016, I called the supervisor of the Division of Nursing Care Facilities in the state capital, Harrisburg, to ask if procedures had changed. She said that investigation procedures were established by the Centers for Medicare & Medicaid Services (CMS); they were still essentially the same; and that it would be difficult to go back to determine why the "no actual harm" code had been assigned in Mary Regina's case in 2012.

CMS does provide a detailed policy manual for the conduct of investigations. However, the manual states the timing, scope, duration, and conduct of a complaint investigation are at the discretion of the State Agency. (CMS guidance is discussed in Chapter 13.)

I was grateful that DOH had cited MRNH on the dehydration issue. If DOH had not, MRNH probably would not have been held accountable for anything at all. Similarly, if I had not filed my complaint, MRNH would not have been held accountable. However, I believe the DOH investigation was neither adequate nor satisfactory.

Chapter 9: The Pennsylvania Department of Health

Over time, before and after I spoke with the supervisor in Harrisburg, I wrote to the Pennsylvania secretary of health, the Pennsylvania auditor general, Pennsylvania Senator Robert P. Casey Jr., the Pennsylvania attorney general, both the state and U.S. Department of Health and Human Services inspectors general, the U.S. Government Accountability Office, and CMS to make officials aware of the oversight results in my mother's case, and to determine whether anything had changed regarding oversight practices.

I ultimately hand-delivered draft copies of the manuscript of this book to the Capitol Hill office of then-President-Elect Trump's nominee for Secretary of Health and Human Services, Congressman Tom Price, and to selected other members of Congress. I sent summaries to Casey, and Speaker of the U.S. House of Representatives Paul Ryan.

I found that a new Pennsylvania secretary of health, Dr. Karen Murphy, PhD, had been appointed by Governor Tom Wolf and confirmed in May 2015. She proved to be among the more responsive government officials to whom I posed questions. She said on March 1, 2016, in response to a February 29 letter from me, "As you may know, I too am very interested in the quality of nursing home care in Pennsylvania. I've taken several steps to improve the quality of health care and quality of life for nursing home residents. I will develop a response to your questions and also share with you the steps that we have taken to achieve our goals."

Statistics that Dr. Murphy provided regarding oversight of nursing homes in Pennsylvania by the Pennsylvania DOH, DNCF, Bureau of Facility Licensure and Certification, mirrored my memory of the insufficiency

Chapter 9: The Pennsylvania Department of Health

of action I had witnessed personally regarding my complaint about my mother.

Enforcement actions had been on a general downward trend since 2003 and more recent annual totals of enforcement actions were small fractions of what they had once been, according to data the DOH provided to me in 2016.

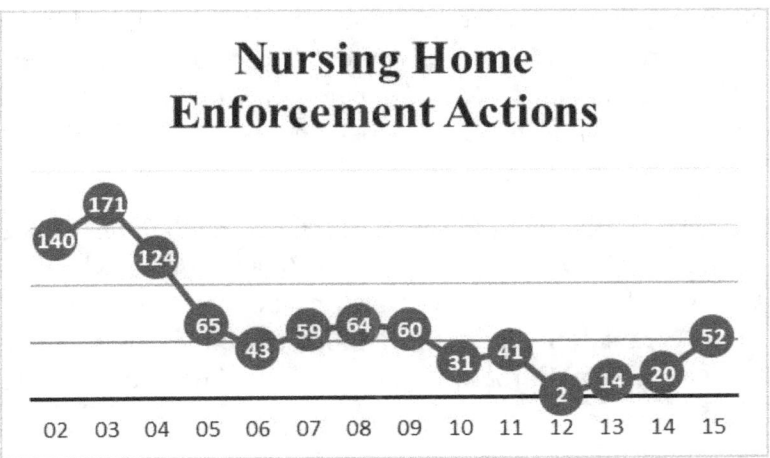

Enforcement actions included, in order of frequency, civil monetary penalties, conversion of regular licenses to provisional licenses, bans on admission, license revocations, and federal terminations of participation in Medicare and Medicaid. The data points on the preceding chart reflect total actions of all types per year.

The average number of enforcement actions for the entire period 2002-2015 was 63.5 per year and the average for the peak 3 years, 2002-2004, was 145 per year. In the single highest year, 2003, 171 total actions were taken, consisting of 89 civil monetary penalties, 74 provisional licenses, seven bans on admission, and one license

Chapter 9: The Pennsylvania Department of Health

revocation. In the year with the fewest enforcement actions, 2012, only two actions of any kind were taken.

Because the 2012 number was so incredibly low, I asked a staffer from the health secretary's office to confirm its accuracy via email, and she did. Notably, 2012 is the year the department investigated my complaint about the treatment of Mary Regina, when DOH coded the lone citation it issued in her case as "No Actual Harm." For 2012, two licenses were converted to provisional, and there were zeros reported in all other enforcement categories. The 2012 statistics seemed consistent with my first-hand experience with the unresponsiveness of the DOH that year.

The 3 years with the fewest enforcement actions in the period 2002-2015 were 2012, 2013, and 2014, when an average of 12 enforcement actions per year were taken. These years fell under the administration of Republican Governor Tom Corbett, Jr. (January 18, 2011-January 20, 2015).

Nursing home industry lobbyists argue that the number of enforcement actions drops as quality of care improves. However, that contention seems questionable, since, in Pennsylvania as well as nationally, as the number of enforcement actions was declining, the number of consumer complaints was rising. This is discussed in Chapter 13.

The number of enforcement actions in Pennsylvania increased 150 percent for 2015 over 2014, coinciding with the appointment of the new secretary of health, Dr. Murphy, and a highly publicized lawsuit by the state attorney general, discussed in Chapter 10, which was filed on July 1, 2015. The 54 enforcement actions in 2015 compared with 20 for 2014. The number of provisional licenses increased 100 percent and civil monetary penalties increased nearly 200 percent year over year, DOH said.

Complaint handling in 2015 also showed notable changes. Partly because the Health Department reinstated the policy of accepting anonymous complaints, it took in 662 more complaints than the previous year.

Complaint Handling by Pennsylvania DOH				
Year	2012	2013	2014	2015
Complaints Received	1,843	1,855	1,930	2,592
Complaints Substantiated	368	446	488	879
Substantiation Rate	20%	24%	25%	34%

The rate of complaint substantiation under Secretary Murphy in 2015 was 34 percent, compared to 20 percent in 2012 and 25 percent in 2014. The preceding table also reflects a 34 percent increase in the number of complaints recorded from 2014 to 2015.

In June 2017, I invited former Governor Corbett to comment on enforcement statistics for his administration and on an allegation by the state auditor general that the Corbett Administration stopped taking anonymous complaints to "silence critics." (That allegation is discussed in more detail in Chapter 11, along with comments by the

Chapter 9: The Pennsylvania Department of Health

auditor general about the adequacy of monetary penalties during part of the Corbett administration.)

Governor Corbett's spokesman, Kevin Harley, provided the following statement:

"Pennsylvania has more than 700 nursing facilities with 88,000 beds and an average of 91 percent capacity with 80,000 patients. The career employees in the Department of Health, whether in the Corbett or Wolf administrations, are dedicated to ensuring nursing home residents are receiving appropriate care.

"It is not unusual for private organizations or politicians with their own economic or political agendas to call into question each administration's motivations in nursing home oversight. The Corbett Administration rejects any characterization by these groups that enforcement was lacking.

"In fact, the Corbett Administration worked with industry and community organizations to improve the reporting of investigations as well as complaint and event reporting. They put in place policies that made sure the information was well documented and accurate. They did not prevent or inhibit reporting but simply changed the format in which the reports, whether they were complaints or events, were received.

"Specifically as it relates to complaints, if an individual submits a complaint it is always confidential unless they request it not to be, so this change in reporting does not have any influence on the amount of complaints received. The decision to prohibit anonymous complaints was intended to improve reporting to allow the inspectors to investigate real and substantive issues, not personnel complaints or HR [human resources] issues that were commonly received through anonymous means. When a complaint is received, the routine practice is to call the complainant and ask for additional information, as most did not provide enough information to investigate the issues thoroughly and appropriately.

"Furthermore, DOH investigated complaints and took actions, if warranted and appropriate. DOH career employees, regardless of administration, take the job of investigating complaints very seriously. There were increases in the number of complaints and complaints substantiated increased in both 2013 and 2014. The same can be said of increases in 2013 and 2014 with the most significant punitive regulatory actions that can be taken by state governments, Civil Monetary Penalties and Provisional Licensure.

"As it relates to fines, there was a steady decline in monetary penalties for more than a decade. It is worth noting this is a question nationally as well. The Government Accounting Office published a report in October 2015 which 'identifies that in recent years, trends in four key sets of data that give insight into nursing home quality show mixed results, and data issues complicate the ability to assess quality trends. Nationally, one of the four data sets -- consumer complaints -- suggests that consumers' concerns over quality have increased, while the other three data sets—deficiencies, staffing levels, and clinical quality measures—indicate potential improvement in nursing home quality.' As you noted, the average number of consumer complaints reported per home increased by 21 percent from 2005-2014, indicating a potential decrease in quality. Conversely, the number of serious deficiencies identified per home with an on-site survey, referred to as a standard survey, decreased by 41 percent over the same period, indicating potential improvement."

Chapter 9: The Pennsylvania Department of Health

I submitted a follow-up question to Harley asking explicitly why the number of enforcement actions fell to two in 2012, but I had not received a reply in time for publication. If I receive one I will post it on my website: https://www.wbeerman.com.

* * *

In August 2015, the DOH established a Nursing Home Quality Improvement Task Force that included five nationally recognized experts in long-term care management from academia, two physicians, and two Pennsylvania legislators. Its objective was to identify areas in which the department's oversight could improve.

The report of the task force is discussed in detail in Chapter 14. Briefly, it called for "effective collaboration between and among government agencies and policy makers, long-term care providers, health care professionals and consumers of long-term care." Although the Task Force commissioned a survey of nursing home residents and included in its report the results of the survey, an October 2016 news release that the DOH issued about the report did not mention the resident survey results at all.

I was disappointed that the results of the resident survey were not widely reported, and I decided to include the survey results in this book. I wanted to provide more attention for the voices of the residents who participated in the survey.

The first question for the survey was, "How satisfied are you with the quality of the physical care provided?" Sixty-two percent of respondents answered "Very dissatisfied."

Chapter 9: The Pennsylvania Department of Health

During her first year in office, after the filing of the attorney general's lawsuit, Secretary Murphy asked State Auditor General Eugene A. DePasquale to audit the policies and procedures pertaining to nursing home complaint management. The audit is discussed in Chapter 11.

Accomplishments during her first year cited by Murphy included:

- Resuming acceptance of anonymous complaints.
- Revising the quality-assurance complaint intake process.
- Reassigning qualified surveyor staff and hiring staff to handle nursing home surveys and complaint investigations.
- Instituting mandatory training and retraining of staff on the compliance process and the determination of scope and severity codes.
- Installing a new system to enhance complaint operations.
- Expanding collaboration with the Department of Aging on survey findings and complaints indicating involvement by Older American Protective Services and Ombudsmen.

Under the administration of Murphy, the DOH increased staffing of the Division of Nursing Care Facilities from 133 to 146, according to the DOH. In 2014 the division's staffing levels were 13 supervisors, 109 Health Facility Quality Examiners (HFQEs), one HFQE trainee, and 10 HFQE vacancies. In August 2016 there were 13 supervisors, 114 HFQEs, six HFQE trainees, seven rehired annuitants, and six HFQE vacancies.

Chapter 9: The Pennsylvania Department of Health

In August 2016, PennLive.com/the *Patriot-News*, in Mechanicsburg, PA, near the state capital of Harrisburg, published a three-article series entitled, "Failing the Frail." The articles contended that the Pennsylvania Department of Health's oversight of nursing homes had been lax.

The articles, written by Daniel Simmons-Ritchie and David Wenner, reported that a 6-month investigation by the news organization concluded that the state's response was insufficient regarding 46 people -- and maybe more – who died due to care-related failures in Pennsylvania nursing homes from 2013 to 2015.

The detailed articles were the result of reviews of hundreds of inspection reports and interviews with more than 60 experts, advocates, government and industry officials, and families of nursing home residents. The information in the articles was consistent with my memories of my mother's nursing home experience and the state's response to my complaints. The articles reinforced my perception that government oversight of nursing homes was unsatisfactory.

The articles quoted critics who said "lax state oversight has allowed nursing homes to put profit over care."

Simmons-Ritchie and Wenner said that the 46 cases in which the Department of Health cited a nursing home for a care-related death were only a fraction of the 259 deaths due to serious incidents that nursing homes reported during the period covered by the articles. The articles further reported that of the 46 cases in which nursing homes were cited, the state decided that penalties were unnecessary in more than half of the cases. When penalties were assessed, the average fine for a care-related death during 2013-2015 was only $13,593.

Chapter 9: The Pennsylvania Department of Health

The PennLive stories said the DOH "appears to consistently understate the severity of death-related cases." The articles said that of the 46 death cases, only one was classified as "immediate jeopardy" – the highest category of severity for an individual occurrence that does not involve a pattern or is not widespread in scope (Code J in the chart in Chapter 13).

The authors added: "But especially concerning to experts interviewed by PennLive is that the department gave seven of the 46 care-related deaths the second lowest severity level, typically known as 'minimal harm'."

The articles quoted Sam Brooks, an attorney with Community Legal Services Philadelphia, who said inspectors often fail to substantiate cases he feels are valid. "He believes, at its root, the department has developed a culture in which inspectors rely too heavily on the testimony of nursing home managers over other evidence." This was a core issue in my 2012 complaint about the DOH's handling of Mary Regina's case.

In a published reader response to the PennLive articles, someone identifying themselves as psu1969 wrote:

Great article! What is sad is that the nursing homes noted as poor care givers have been problematic for decades. The problem as I see it is multifaceted. Extra training for CNAs (Certified Nurse's Aides) is the tip of the iceberg. State inspectors need to be trained better, DOH consistency from field office to field office needs to be imposed, federal oversight of DOH needs to be enhanced and politics needs to be removed from the equation. Nursing home corporations need to be held accountable for the games they play relative to regulations....

If you have a loved one in a nursing home you must be their advocate, because the Department of Health is really deficient on that front.

Chapter 10: The New Mexico and Pennsylvania Attorneys General; Controversial Lawsuits; a Pornography Scandal; and a Jail Sentence

I found that lawsuits filed by state attorneys general (AGs) against chains of nursing homes operating in their states provide valuable and unsurpassed insight into the world of nursing homes. This is true whether, or not, the defendant nursing homes ultimately are found to be guilty and liable for wrongdoing.

The process for the AG lawsuits not only includes investigation of the treatment of the nursing home residents, but it also probes into the corporate structures, finances, and operations of nursing homes and nursing home chains. In addition, the AGs look at the interaction between nursing homes and their government oversight agencies, in some respects.

The four AG lawsuits that I focused on encompassed 65 defendant nursing homes and the care provided during more than a million nursing home patient-days. The suits covered defendant nursing home corporation operations in New Mexico and Pennsylvania, but not operations by nursing homes in other states in which some of the defendant corporations also operated. Conditions alleged are not likely to be unique to New Mexico and Pennsylvania.

The AGs conducted their cases with help from a large Washington, DC law firm. The AG-private law firm collaboration achieved a breadth and depth of investigation that may be unlikely to occur in a suit filed on behalf of one individual nursing home resident against one nursing home. However, Appendix D has an interesting perspective on nursing home lawsuits undertaken by private attorneys.

I learned the following from AG lawsuits; these are just a few examples.

- A considerable number of nursing homes knew in advance when state inspectors were coming for "unannounced" government inspections.

- The gap between the services promised and paid for and the services actually delivered was quantifiable using scientific stopwatch and computer simulation methods. For one defendant nursing home chain, the New Mexico AG alleged that the hours of care provided fell short of patient needs by quantities ranging from 20.4 percent to 70.0 percent during various calendar quarters at various nursing homes.

- The staffing cost for a nursing home might be lower if the staff keeps a resident in diapers or incontinence briefs, even if the resident is not incontinent, because it takes less time to change a

Chapter 10: The Attorney General Lawsuits

resident than it does to respond to a resident's call for help to get to the toilet.

- Even lawyers wielding the power of the state AG offices can face formidable challenges in obtaining information from defendant nursing home corporations. Defendants said they simply did not have records demanded by the attorney general; they could not produce critical records because a hacker had launched a "ransomware" attack against the chain's computer system; and that email records were at least temporarily inaccessible because of a computer crash.

    o At a February 21, 2017 hearing, when defense lawyers said their clients had no records about transfers of profits among corporate entities or individuals, New Mexico Judge Sara Singleton commented, "I mean, unless they are passing this money around in paper bags, it is really hard to believe there is not some record of it somewhere." A defense lawyer responded, "Your Honor, I can only report to you what I have received from my client." He added, "I'm happy to go back and further explore this with my clients, your Honor." The judge told him she thought he should do that.

    o After expressing concern that nursing homes may not have provided a backup system for their records, Judge Singleton said to a defense attorney: "So we are going to fight later about whether there was sufficient precaution on your part, or whether some sort of spoliation inference or claim can be made. . . ." In New

Chapter 10: The Attorney General Lawsuits

Mexico, "spoliation" in a legal sense can refer to destruction of evidence to defeat a lawsuit.

- Lawsuits were contentious and very complicated, or, as one attorney commented, contain "lots of moving parts." One hearing in Santa Fe had seven lawyers present in the courtroom to argue over arcane points of law. A suit about nursing home care can be challenged and possibly dismissed over a technicality that has nothing to do with nursing homes per se, resident care, or the core allegations of the case.

I have posted some detailed lawsuit documents including complaints and court decisions on my website at https://www.wbeerman.com for readers who may have time to peruse them.

In December 2014, New Mexico AG Gary King filed suit against seven nursing homes operated in the state at various times by the Preferred Care or Cathedral Rock chains. The suit alleged the homes and, in some cases, certain affiliated corporations located out of state, violated the state's Fraud Against Taxpayers Act, its Medicaid Fraud Act, and its Unfair Practices Act. The suit claimed the difference between the services the defendants actually provided and the services they claimed to provide was "profound."

AG Hector Balderas continued the case after he succeeded King in January 2015, along with Patricia Padrino Tucker, the deputy director of the Medicaid Fraud and Elder Abuse Division of the Office of the AG.

The New Mexico suit relied heavily on "widely accepted" scientific "stopwatch" studies and computer simulation modeling of how much time was necessary to perform nursing home care tasks. The AG compared the results of the studies and modeling with the staff sizes of the defendant nursing homes.

"Quite basically," said the AG complaint, "if residents require 250 hours of care each day, but a nursing facility only has enough CNAs (certified nurse's aides) to provide 125 hours of care, it will be unable to provide the care required."

As an example of quantifying the time required for tasks, the lawsuit complaint cited data for the tasks of simultaneously providing required periodic repositioning of a resident while performing incontinence care (changing a diaper or briefs, wet clothing, and linens), which are often done together. According to scientific studies, the two tasks required a minimum of 3 minutes, a maximum of 8 minutes, and a mode (most often) of 5.5 minutes. The suit said the combined activity of repositioning and toileting takes longer: a minimum of 5 minutes, a maximum of 10 minutes, and a mode of 7.5 minutes.

I observed that this could be a reason that staff in some nursing homes might not rush to respond to calls from residents asking for help getting to the bathroom.

The New Mexico AG obtained from the Centers for Medicare & Medicaid Services (CMS) quarterly records from 2008-2014 showing what services the nursing homes had claimed were needed for each of their residents. The suit alleged that, with the staffs the nursing homes had, it was physically and mathematically impossible for nursing homes to perform all of the tasks for which the nursing homes billed Medicaid and private payers. The AG supported the math computations with statements by

Chapter 10: The Attorney General Lawsuits

confidential eyewitnesses who told of alleged neglect in nursing homes.

"Defendants' staffing practices saved them the cost of labor but cost residents their dignity and comfort, and jeopardized their safety," the New Mexico suit said.

The lawsuit complaint presented, for each defendant nursing home, a chart showing quarterly "omissions" of basic care that ranged in certain categories from 20 percent to 70 percent of the services needed. Home-by-home descriptions of the alleged prevailing conditions covered 65 pages of the 134-page lawsuit complaint.

During pre-trial hearings, defendants' attorneys argued that the laws under which the nursing homes were accused dealt with making false statements or claims. The attorneys said the state's complaint had not shown the defendants had lied, even if there were deficiencies in care. The billing procedures for Medicaid, which were based on the number of patients per day, did not require that bills explicitly detail the care provided to obtain payment, the defendants' attorneys contended. One attorney argued that a failure to provide enough care is not the equivalent of lying about the care that was provided.

The defendants also argued that the state's witnesses who described neglect of residents should be viewed in the context of "hundreds or thousands of residents at those facilities."

Further, the defendants argued that because the nursing homes were regulated by state and federal agencies, which together had a complete system of regulations and penalties, it was inappropriate for the AG to file its own lawsuit. They pointed out that the AG lawsuit, with private

Chapter 10: The Attorney General Lawsuits

counsel assisting, could result in a substantial fee award (to be paid by the defendants) to the private law firm. The defendants argued that the regulatory system recognizes that there will be lapses in care and that the existing system is designed to deal with those lapses with fines and other sanctions imposed by the health department and/or the federal government. Regulation by the health department does not involve legal fees, the defendants pointed out.

The defendants also contended that the stop watch and computer simulations had never been used by the New Mexico Department of Health and that those methods amounted to applying new standards retroactively for the defendants.

The AG countered by contending that simply by billing for services that they had not provided, the nursing homes were in effect lying to obtain payment, and violating applicable laws.

The New Mexico Preferred Care suit was scheduled for a status hearing before Judge David Thompson on September 27, 2018. The results will be reported on the website wbeerman.com. Proceedings in the state court had been stayed pending legal determinations in bankruptcy court. A statement issued by Preferred Care, Inc., of Plano, Texas, said it filed Chapter 11 bankruptcy proceedings in November 2017 to allow it to remain in business as it defended against 163 personal injury cases.

In Pennsylvania, on July 1, 2015, former Pennsylvania AG Kathleen G. Kane, and Thomas M. Devlin, chief deputy AG for the Health Care Section, Public Protection Division, of the Office of the Attorney General (OAG), filed a legal action against 14 Pennsylvania nursing homes in the Golden Living nursing home chain (a different chain

Chapter 10: The Attorney General Lawsuits

from the one involved in Mary Regina's case in Pennsylvania). It covered the chain's practices from 2008-2014. After the initial news coverage, the suit grew to encompass 25 of Golden's 36 nursing homes in Pennsylvania, as 350 complaints were submitted and 11 nursing homes were added to the suit on September 9, 2015.

In all, since 2015, three Pennsylvania AG lawsuits made allegations that were similar to those in the New Mexico suit, but did not use scientific stopwatch studies. The Pennsylvania AG did, for its part, have much more financial information about the nursing homes than the New Mexico AG had acquired for its suit by the time this book was published.

The Pennsylvania Golden Living suit was dismissed by the state's Commonwealth Court on March 22, 2017, but was pending an appeal in the Pennsylvania Supreme Court as of July 2018. Appendix C provides a summary outline of the reasons for dismissal cited by the Commonwealth Court, along with a brief summary of a judge's dissenting opinion in the case. The entire Commonwealth Court decision is on my website at https://www.wbeerman.com, along with various other court documents including any subsequent decisions on appeals.

One Pennsylvania AG nursing home suit, filed against the Reliant Senior Care Holdings chain, was settled in October 2016, with Reliant agreeing in a consent decree to pay $2 million to the state. The settlement said, "This Consent Decree is made in compromise of the Parties' dispute. This Consent Decree is neither an admission of liability by Reliant nor a concession by the Attorney General that its claims are not well-founded." The settlement includes an injunction prohibiting Reliant from

Chapter 10: The Attorney General Lawsuits

violating the Pennsylvania Consumer Protection Law in specified ways and requires quality-of-care improvements. The AG said Reliant cooperated with the AG's investigation.

Reliant operated 22 skilled nursing facilities in Pennsylvania. The suit alleged that Reliant limited the number of CNAs, rendering the facilities incapable of delivering the basic care that residents were promised and needed. The disposition of the $2 million and the fees paid to a private law firm are discussed later in this chapter.

A third Pennsylvania AG nursing home lawsuit was filed on November 3, 2016 against Grane Healthcare and 11 of its nursing homes. It had key similarities with the other Pennsylvania suits and one of its attorneys told a newspaper that Grane would file objections that were generally similar to those that led to the Commonwealth Court's dismissal of the Golden Living case.

On May 11, 2017, Commonwealth Court approved discontinuance of the Grane case and ultimate withdrawal of the complaint against the defendants, in the aftermath of the dismissal of the Golden Living case and Supreme Court consideration of an appeal of the dismissal. The Commonwealth Court approved withdrawal "without prejudice" and the case conceivably could be re-filed at a later time.

In the Grane case, the AG alleged the following:

"The Grane Facilities had the resources to pay for increased staffing levels -- either increased payroll for regular employees or the cost of temporary staffing services. However, instead of providing adequate staffing to meet the needs of residents, they diverted significant

Chapter 10: The Attorney General Lawsuits

amounts of profit each year to their owners in ways that made the facilities appear less profitable than they really were. For example, Grane Facilities entered into lease agreements with related companies (owned by the same owners) that owned the real property on which each facility was located, agreeing to pay in rent each year a particular base rent *plus any profit that the facility made over the year.*

"These agreements resulted in a significant transfer of assets -- millions of dollars each year -- from the Grane Facilities to the entities that owned the property which were, in turn, owned by the same people who owned the Grane Facilities. The transfers of assets through these lease agreements allowed the Grane Facilities to report little or no profit on cost reports submitted to the Pennsylvania Medical Assistance Program. In sum, a significant amount of the revenue received by the Grane Facilities -- money paid by the Pennsylvania Medical Assistance Program and by Pennsylvania consumers for resident care -- was diverted out of the Grane Facilities, rather than used to pay for the staffing levels the facilities needed to provide adequate care to residents."

A controversial aspect that the AG cases had in common was the AGs' collaboration in the suits with a private law firm known for suing nursing home chains and for filing other class action suits in cooperation with state AGs. Signing on to the Golden Living suit along with AG attorneys Kane and Devlin were attorneys Victoria S. Nugent and Johanna M. Hickman of the Washington D.C. law firm of Cohen Milstein Sellers & Toll. Nugent and Hickman also were participants in the Reliant and Grane

Chapter 10: The Attorney General Lawsuits

cases and were admitted to practice in the New Mexico courts to participate in the New Mexico Preferred Care/Cathedral Rock lawsuit.

Defendants alleged in nationally publicized news stories that the Cohen Milstein law firm made campaign contributions to AGs, instigated the AGs to file lawsuits to generate fees for the firm, and made claims in lawsuits about problems that did not exist. AG responses to such claims are discussed later.

A separate, loosely related, interesting aspect of the Golden Living case involved AG Kathleen Kane herself, particularly her high news profile and her political battles, which highlighted the involvement of politics in the Pennsylvania AG office and to some extent among state Supreme Court justices. Kane exposed an email network that had passed graphic pornography and sexist and racist jokes among state employees, including in law enforcement and judicial offices. News reports said the scandal led two Pennsylvania Supreme Court justices to be suspended and then resign. The scandal was reported even by the London *Daily Mail*.

News reports also described political infighting among specific individual Supreme Court justices.

At least one news report said that among those implicated in the porn network were staffers who worked in the AG's office under Republican former AG Tom Corbett before Kane took over as AG. Two of the Corbett staffers in the email scandal eventually served in the governor's cabinet after Corbett was elected governor.

The scandal was called "The Great Pennsylvania Government Porn Caper" in a February 24, 2016 *Esquire*

Chapter 10: The Attorney General Lawsuits

article by journalist David Gambacorta, who referred to the state's capital as "the nerve center of its incestuous, dysfunctional political system."

Kane's opponents accused her of stifling prosecution of Philadelphia Democrat politicians that had been started by her Republican predecessor, and she ultimately was charged and convicted of perjury and of releasing secret grand jury information in an attempt to discredit a political enemy.

Kane, a Democrat, said she was up against "trumped up charges" and a "good old boys" culture.

On March 16, 2016, a Common Pleas Court judge sentenced Kane to 10-23 months of jail time.

About a year later, the Pennsylvania Commonwealth Court threw out Kane's Golden Living nursing home lawsuit. The appeal of the Golden Living case went to the Pennsylvania Supreme Court, which, as noted, had lost two of its justices as a result of Kane's pornography expose'.

I found in news archives no reporting about a connection between the Golden Living nursing home case and Kane's role in the email scandal, the Supreme Court resignations, or Pennsylvania politics. But the story illustrated the fact that politicians do play a role in decision making about nursing homes. Another example is that Democrat Pennsylvania Auditor General Eugene DePasquale strongly criticized, in an audit report, the administration of former Republican Governor Corbett (January 18, 2011 to January 20, 2015) for banning anonymous complaints about nursing homes. This is discussed in Chapter 11.

Chapter 10: The Attorney General Lawsuits

Regarding links between politics and the nursing home industry, I thought it was interesting that the president and CEO of the American Health Care Association (AHCA) and National Center for Assisted Living, the nation's largest association of long-term and post-acute care providers, is Mark Parkinson, the former governor of Kansas. He was an elder care facilities developer, and the running mate and lieutenant governor under Governor Kathleen Sebelius, who subsequently served as secretary of the U.S. Department of Health and Human Services (HHS) from April 28, 2009 to June 9, 2014 under President Obama. HHS is the parent agency of CMS, which oversees nursing homes at the federal level.

On June 12, 2017, Parkinson appeared along with other nursing home industry officials in a news release photo taken at HHS with new HHS Secretary Tom Price.

In essence, the Golden Living suit accused nursing home companies associated with Golden Living of misleading the government and private consumers, who together paid the nursing homes' bills, by promising and charging for basic services, but failing to provide all of the services. The suit alleged violations of the state's Unfair Trade Practices and Consumer Protection Law (UTPCPL) and contended nursing home staffing was insufficient to provide the promised services to residents.

The lawsuit focused public scrutiny on conditions in Pennsylvania nursing homes by citing accounts of nursing home life by confidential witnesses and by recounting the homes' histories of health department citations.

Something contained in Attorney General Kane's Golden Living lawsuit complaint reminded me of the

Chapter 10: The Attorney General Lawsuits

reason I decided a half-century earlier, in 1966, to go to journalism school and become a newspaper reporter.

That something was a single sentence I read on page 145 as I browsed through the 216-page lawsuit complaint.

The sentence said: "**Managers knew when DOH (Department of Health) inspections were coming, and they would rush to make sure everything was set for the inspection.**"

I then read the entire lawsuit document, and counted statements in which 13 confidential witnesses – mostly former nursing home employees – from 11 different nursing homes in the 36-nursing-home Pennsylvania Golden Living chain -- told the OAG in essence that nursing homes knew that DOH was coming before surveyors (inspectors) arrived for "unannounced" inspections.

One witness, a CNA who worked at a Golden Living facility from 2009-2012, said he normally was responsible for as many as 15 residents on morning and evening shifts, and as many as 23 on night shifts. The lawsuit quoted him as follows:

"Administrators knew ahead of time when a DOH inspection was about to take place. They would hold a meeting right before each inspection and say that they had heard the facility would be inspected in a few days and that the staff should get the facility clean. On inspection days, everything was clean and perfect, everyone was helpful, and supplies were fully stocked. The Administrator would even put out new socks for the residents. There were also more staff on inspection days. The facility would bring in CNAs who were part-time or who usually worked other

Chapter 10: The Attorney General Lawsuits

shifts. Because everyone helped out on inspection days, the CNAs would only have to be responsible for about 7-8 residents each."

Another confidential witness said: "Management knew when DOH surveyors were coming. Employees with office jobs would come out of their offices to help on the floor on inspection days .... **the State did not get an accurate picture of real life at the facility**."

Real life at the nursing homes was portrayed in the Golden Living lawsuit, through statements of confidential witnesses, including family members, and reports from DOH surveyors, as appalling. The suit summarized, "Golden Living Facilities were so understaffed that residents were thirsty, hungry, dirty and unkempt, and found that when they tried to summon help, no one was available to meet their most basic needs, like escorting them to a toilet or refilling a water glass."

The lawsuit did not mention the fact that federal regulations require that surveys be unannounced.

The federal government's (CMS's) State Operations Manual, Appendix P – Survey Protocol for Long-Term Care Facilities, is a policy and procedures manual for state nursing home oversight agencies, such as the Pennsylvania Health Department. It details how inspectors should conduct surveys (inspections) of skilled nursing facilities (SNFs) and nursing facilities (NFs).

Appendix P directs up front in the Introduction section: "**Do not announce SNF/NF Surveys to the facility**."

Manual Paragraph 5300 -- Investigation of Complaints for Nursing Homes, states: "**Onsite complaint investigations should always be unannounced**." (5300.2)

Chapter 10: The Attorney General Lawsuits

I queried CMS about this and Karen Tritz, director, Division of Nursing Homes, Survey and Certification Group, provided the following information.

The policies in the manual and appendices are derived from federal law: 42 Code of Federal Regulations, Paragraph 488.307. Subparagraph (a) states, "All standard surveys must be unannounced." Subparagraph (b) states that CMS is to review scheduling and surveying practices to ensure survey agencies [such as Pennsylvania DOH] avoid giving notice of a survey through scheduling procedures and the conduct of the surveys. Subparagraph (b) (2) states that CMS is to take corrective action if agencies are found to have notified nursing homes of surveys through scheduling or procedural policies, and agencies are subject to sanctions if they are found to have notified nursing homes in advance of surveys.

Subparagraph (c) states: "An individual who notifies a SNF or NF, or causes a SNF or NF to be notified, of the time or date on which a standard survey is to be conducted is subject to a Federal civil monetary penalty not to exceed $2,000."

I thought back to my days as a teenager in the 1960s when I hung out in a pool hall on East Fifth Avenue in McKeesport, PA. Patrons in the pool hall knew in advance when the Allegheny County racket squad was going to raid the illegal gambling (numbers racket) joints and the Brick Alley prostitution houses in town.

I was fascinated. "How do people know about the raids in advance?" I wondered. "How does this stuff work?"

Curiosity about such matters was a big reason I decided to become a newspaper reporter.

Chapter 10: The Attorney General Lawsuits

After journalism school, as a green cub reporter for the *New Pittsburgh Courier*, I was given an opportunity to pursue my interest in organized crime. The *Courier*'s executive editor, the late Carl E. Morris, gave me a tip that the United States attorney for the Western District of Pennsylvania, Richard L. Thornburgh, was going to indict the Allegheny County district attorney and the chief of the county detectives' racket squad.

Top county officials who were supposed to be enforcing the law allegedly were breaking it by protecting the racketeers, and possibly getting payoffs.

Some might recognize the name of Thornburgh because he would eventually become governor of Pennsylvania and the attorney general of the United States.

I went to the Federal Building or to the U.S. Courthouse -- I can't remember which it was -- to interview Thornburgh. I do remember distinctly how Thornburgh's secretary announced me. "The *Courier* is here to see you," she said. I had never been called "The *Courier*" before. I thought I was now in the big leagues of newspaper reporting. I was then admitted to the U.S. attorney's personal office. As an unsophisticated 21-year-old, I was impressed by the ambiance: the huge executive desk, leather chairs for visitors, a conference table, and an American flag behind Thornburgh's desk. I am not sure, but I think there was some sort of U.S. Department of Justice seal, either on a wall or on a carpet. After posing my questions to Thornburgh, I went to interview the two alleged targets of the investigation in a nearby county building.

After the interviews, which were quite brief, I told Carl Morris that Thornburgh had declined to comment, and that

Chapter 10: The Attorney General Lawsuits

the district attorney and the chief of the county detectives' racket squad both denied knowing anything at all about any investigation.

I told Morris, "You must have gotten a bad tip." It was a colossally stupid, naïve, conclusion and probably the worst mistake I would make in my news reporting career, which then was only about a year old. I am amazed that Morris did not fire me and I now admire him for granting me clemency.

Thornburgh did obtain an indictment of the district attorney for failing to report income. The DA, Robert W. Duggan, who was married to a well-known heiress, was found at his farm dead of a mysterious shotgun wound hours before a federal grand jury indicted him. It probably was the biggest political story ever to happen in Pittsburgh.

The county detectives most likely were the sources of the pool hall patrons' advance information about the raids on the bookies and prostitutes. Of course, if the guys at the pool hall knew, so did the racketeers and pimps, and many other people in town. The raids were largely for show, and business as usual would resume after the raids. The raids were a joke.

I found out about racketeering in Allegheny County in a humiliating way that did not enhance my newspaper career prospects. But the experience made the statement, **"Managers knew when DOH inspections were coming,"** jump out of that nursing home lawsuit document for me. I knew the significance: it was a red flag for possible corruption, just like the advance knowledge that the county detectives were coming to town for a "raid."

Chapter 10: The Attorney General Lawsuits

Maybe nursing home managers were just good guessers about when the surveyors/inspectors would come and maybe there were predictors, such as approaching deadlines. If a survey was supposed to be done annually, and the annual "survey window" was coming to a close, nursing home managers might be confident that a survey was imminent. Or maybe managers would find out that the inspectors were at the nursing home down the street, and figured they were next. Maybe nobody from DOH was tipping off the nursing homes.

Nevertheless, I thought, if surveys/inspections are supposed to review normal operations, surveyors should make sure they do the survey when operations are normal, not after a nursing home has temporarily augmented and rallied its staff to prepare.

Pennsylvania was not the only state where a nursing home might know about an inspection in advance. The New Mexico AG nursing home lawsuit also mentioned a nursing home knowing in advance of impending inspections, and the knowledge allegedly went all the way up to the home's corporate office. A lawsuit document quoted a confidential witness as saying:

"*Casa Real* (nursing home) took steps to hide its typical conditions and staffing from DOH. The Cathedral Rock corporate office knew DOH surveyors were coming ahead of time and would conduct a preliminary survey in advance. They would reach full staffing levels for surveys by calling all of the CNAs in – even those who were not scheduled to work. The food even looked better during surveys."

I viewed the allegations that nursing homes knew when inspectors were coming in the context of the

Chapter 10: The Attorney General Lawsuits

Pennsylvania DOH's attempts to blow off my own complaints about my mother's care in 2012. I wondered whether the DOH had been (1) passively lax or incompetent, (2) too rushed, or (3) actively protecting the nursing homes when it investigated complaints.

When I asked about the allegations in the Pennsylvania attorney general's lawsuit concerning advance knowledge of survey timing by nursing homes, a spokesperson for the Pennsylvania secretary of health said:

"The department is required to survey each facility with a 12- to 16-month window in order to meet state and federal requirements. The department very conscientiously ensures that survey schedules are not disclosed to facilities and makes every effort to vary the timing of surveys to minimize the 'predictability' of the next one. The department is not aware of information about survey schedules or timing being disclosed to facilities."

Nevertheless, at least during the time covered by the lawsuit, 2008-2013, 11 different Pennsylvania nursing homes in one chain, and others in Pennsylvania and New Mexico, allegedly knew of inspections in advance, according to the confidential witnesses.

The Pennsylvania state attorney general's office declined to comment about whether it was looking into tip-offs to nursing homes about impending state inspections. It seemed to me that the advance information reported by the confidential witnesses could be traced back to the person who gave the information to them, and up the chain, back to the root source.

I submitted a Freedom of Information Act (FOIA) request to CMS, which oversees nursing homes and the

Chapter 10: The Attorney General Lawsuits

state agencies that inspect them, for information about any sanctions it issued against the Pennsylvania DOH or other state agencies for allowing nursing homes to know about impending inspections, or for poor performance of inspections. I also sent CMS a copy of the complaint in the Golden Living lawsuit, which included the allegations by confidential witnesses. David R. Wright, director of the CMS Center for Clinical Standards and Quality/Survey and Certification Group, responded:

"Regarding the request for sanctions imposed on individuals for advanced notice of surveys: We do not have information on this type of sanction and believe it is overseen by the Office of Inspector General (OIG).

"Regarding the request for statistics on sanctions imposed on States for unsatisfactory survey practices: We do not have statistics on sanctions. However, we note that CMS monitors State survey performance regularly and requires corrective action plans to be implemented to improve performance. Also, we take additional actions when necessary, such as:

- "Benchmarking funding, which requires a State to meet certain thresholds to allow for continued funding; or
- "Setting specific deliverables which, if not met, may result in termination of the [use of that state agency to inspect nursing homes]."

I followed up with an additional request for statistics about benchmarking actions and requests for deliverables and trends concerning unsatisfactory survey practices. I was told to submit Freedom of Information Act requests. I also wrote letters to the U.S. Department of Health and

Chapter 10: The Attorney General Lawsuits

Human Services and Pennsylvania inspectors general about any sanctions they imposed, but I did not receive a response from the IGs before publication of this book.

In a partial, "FOIA SWIFT task" courtesy response to my questions about the Benchmarking, Wright's office said the following, while noting that other information would have to come from regional offices.

"Benchmark funding has been utilized each of the last few years, beginning in FY 2012. This funding methodology has only been utilized to focus on those states which have shown performance issues from the previous FY. If a state is given a benchmark, a set amount of funding is set aside for a particular state until an adequate correction plan is submitted and benchmarks are met .... While the numbers have reduced some, it should be noted that not all of the states receiving benchmarks are repeated from year to year."

CMS said 12 states received benchmarks in fiscal 2012; five in 2013; nine in 2014; eight in 2015; and eight in 2016.

Other information I requested through FOIA requests had not been provided by CMS at the time of publication.

I believed CMS should be able to say in detail what it was doing to ensure state survey agencies were operating effectively and in accordance with CMS regulations, and what it did when they were not, such as when they allowed nursing homes to know in advance about inspections.

I felt this was especially true in light of sensational allegations being made about inadequate oversight of nursing homes by state agencies. A set of five questions I submitted to CMS and HHS just before publication of this

Chapter 10: The Attorney General Lawsuits

book in June 2017, and the CMS reply, are presented in Appendix D.

Shortly after the initial edition of my book was published, a Florida state government oversight official was sentenced in December 2017 to 57 months in prison for selling to nursing home operators advance copies of confidential nursing home inspection schedules and copies of complaints filed by patients. The website, wbeerman.com, has articles about this case in its archives section, including one with a headline, "Yes, at least one nursing home oversight employee did take bribes."

Allegations about normal conditions in the Golden Living nursing homes – at times when the homes were not expecting inspectors – were outlined in a news release issued by former Attorney General Kane. They included:

- Continent residents were left in diapers because they were unable to obtain assistance going to the bathroom.
- Incontinent residents were left in soiled diapers, in their own feces or urine, for extended periods of time.
- Residents were at risk for bedsores from not being turned every 2 hours as required.
- Residents were not receiving range-of-motion exercises.
- Residents were not receiving showers or other hygiene services as required.
- Residents were being awakened at 5 a.m. or earlier to be washed and dressed for the day (because staffing on the day shift was inadequate).
- Residents were not being dressed in time for them to attend their meals.

Chapter 10: The Attorney General Lawsuits

- Residents were not being escorted to the dining hall and sometimes were missing meals entirely.
- There were long waits for responses to call bells or no response at all.
- Staff, under the direction of management or fear of management, falsified records to indicate residents received services when in fact they did not.

Kane also noted that staffing was improved when state inspections occurred, and said that led to deceit about the true conditions at the facility.

The Kane lawsuit investigation also included a review of staffing levels self-reported by Golden Living facilities and deficiencies cited in surveys conducted by the state DOH.

The central argument in the lawsuit was that because of inadequate staffing, the nursing homes did not provide all of the services they promised and for which they were paid.

In response to the lawsuit, Golden Living published on November 16, 2015 a letter signed by 25 of its medical directors in Pennsylvania, affirming their support of their caregiving team and inviting the public to visit their centers to see the care they provide.

In a news story in the *Republican Herald*, Pottsville, PA, Heather Taylor, director of nursing at Golden Living-York Terrace, one of the facilities named in the suit, said the facility was rated five-stars on the federal Five-Star system, meaning it was far above average, and it had a deficiency-free Department of Health score in 2014. The irony of this did not escape me.

Chapter 10: The Attorney General Lawsuits

I was surprised to see one specific Golden Living nursing home included in the suit. When I was trying to get my mother out of her two-star facility in 2011, I attempted to move her to that particular Golden Living facility, which had four stars at the time. Family members and I visited the Golden Living facility twice, and we were favorably impressed.

Golden Living issued a news release in which it said: "Golden Living is confident that claims made by the attorney general are baseless and wholly without merit. No doubt, this is an unfortunate result of Kathleen Kane's inappropriate and questionable relationship with a Washington, DC-based plaintiff's firm that preys on legitimate businesses and is then paid by contingency fees …. We plan to vigorously defend the reputation of Golden Living and its employees."

The attorney general's arrangement with the Washington-based law firm, Cohen Milstein Sellers & Toll, is discussed later in this chapter.

Golden Living said it was a family of companies that specialized in recovery care and that it was a national leader in providing skilled nursing and post-acute care. The companies included Golden Living Centers, Aegis Therapies, AseraCare, and 360 Healthcare Staffing. There were 295 Golden Living Centers in 21 states, the company said.

Golden Living also offered assisted living services in 21 locations, according to a November 2015 news release. In addition, Golden Living said the Golden Living companies provided services to more than 1,000 nursing homes, hospitals, and other healthcare organizations in 41 states and the District of Columbia. Golden said its family

Chapter 10: The Attorney General Lawsuits

of companies had more than 40,000 employees who provided healthcare to 60,000 patients daily.

There was news coverage of the Pennsylvania lawsuit in other states where Golden Living had facilities.

In addition to the individual Golden Living nursing homes, Attorney General Kane sued five different affiliated companies in Plano, TX and Fort Smith, AR: GGNSC (Golden Gate National Senior Care) Holdings (doing business as Golden Horizons), Golden Gate National Senior Care, GGNSC Administrative Services, GGNSC Clinical Services, and GGNSC Equity Holdings. The lawsuit said Golden Horizons directly or indirectly owned each of the Golden Living parent entities as well as each of the Golden Living facilities.

The suit said that between 2008 and 2013 eight Pennsylvania Golden Living facilities each paid total amounts ranging from $256,484 to $363,303 for the period to a company owned by Golden Horizons for home-office administrative costs. During the same period, the same facilities each paid another company owned by Golden Horizons total amounts ranging from $349,972 to $484,078 for administrative, nursing-related, dietary-related, and social service-related costs. Also during the same period, the same facilities each paid another company owned by Golden Gate total amounts ranging from $1.9 million to $2.8 million in administrative costs, according to the lawsuit.

"The Golden Living Facilities are enormously profitable," said the lawsuit. "Payments made by the Golden Living Facilities to the Golden Living Parent Entities provide one mechanism by which the significant profits of the Golden Living Facilities are siphoned out of

Chapter 10: The Attorney General Lawsuits

the facilities and transferred to Golden Horizons, and likely, ultimately, to the ultimate owner of the company: Fillmore Capital Partners."

The lawsuit said that during 2008-2013, profits from 10 Golden Living facilities ranged for the entire period from $1.6 million to $10.4 million individually. Adding the numbers indicates the total profit for the 10 facilities for the 6 years was about $54 million on net revenue of about $546 million.

"These figures reflect the profits as stated in annual cost reports submitted by the facilities to the Commonwealth," the lawsuit said. "However, these calculations of profit do not take into account certain adjustments made to the reported expenses in these cost reports. On information and belief, each facility's true profitability is significantly higher – as much as double the reported profits."

The AG asked the court to require Golden Living to pay civil penalties, restitution, and restoration to the Commonwealth of Pennsylvania and consumers, and court costs. The suit estimated one third of the services paid for were not provided or properly provided, and asked for a judgment in an amount to be determined at trial.

The suit also asked the court to impose civil penalties of up to $1,000 for each violation and $3,000 for each violation involving a person 60 years old or older.

The Washington firm of Cohen Milstein Sellers & Toll teams with state attorneys general in lawsuits against nursing home chains and other business entities. For example, the firm collaborated with New Mexico Attorney General Hector Balderas and his predecessor Gary King to

Chapter 10: The Attorney General Lawsuits

sue seven New Mexico skilled nursing facilities and a management firm serving the facilities.

An April 2015 article by *Legal NewsLine* said Cohen Milstein had donated $71,000 to 16 state attorney general campaigns since 2010. The National Institute on Money in State Politics (NIMSP) reported that the law firm contributed $10,000 to Kane in 2012 and $5,000 to Balderas in 2013. I found through NIMSP that Cohen Milstein also contributed $5,000 to former Pennsylvania Congressman Patrick J. Murphy, who lost to Kane in the 2012 Democratic attorney general primary.

Cohen Milstein's adversary in the Golden Living case also was making campaign contributions, as I found out from the Center for Responsive Politics (CRP). With regard to Federal Election Commission records current as of February 8, 2017, for the 2015-2016 election cycle, CRP reported that Golden Living's national political action committee (PAC) contributed $70,500 to federal candidates, including Pennsylvania Congressmen Dwight Evans ($1,000) and Joe Pitts ($1,000), and Senators Bob Casey ($2,500) and Pat Toomey ($2,500). Also notable was a $10,000 contribution by Golden to Speaker of the House Paul Ryan, who was the Golden PAC's largest recipient among congressmen and senators. NIMSP reported that Golden Living also gave $2,500 to Pennsylvania Senate Pro Tem Joseph B. Scarnati III in 2016.

Nursing home operators filed suit in Pennsylvania Commonwealth Court in an attempt to block the Kane-Cohen Milstein investigation of Pennsylvania nursing homes. They said:

"Cohen Milstein seeks to enrich itself through large contingent fees based on litigation claims made against

Chapter 10: The Attorney General Lawsuits

petitioners in the name of OAG (Office of Attorney General).

"The investigation by Respondent Kane, OAG, and Cohen Milstein was not prompted by any material consumer complaints to OAG for allegedly insufficient care, but rather was initiated by Cohen Milstein to extract legal fee recoveries, as reported in *The New York Times* and other sources." (Eric Lipton did a major story in *The New York Times* on December 18, 2014 on Cohen-Milstein's collaboration with state attorneys general. The headline was "Lawyers Create Big Paydays by Coaxing Attorney Generals to Sue.")

"This Cohen Milstein-driven investigation is an effort to create a 'problem' where none exists in search of profits for itself," said the nursing home operators in their suit.

The suit said the OAG-Cohen Milstein action against the nursing homes was improper and in derogation of the exclusive authority of the Pennsylvania Department of Health.

The challenge was dismissed by Commonwealth Court on January 11, 2016, and the core Kane-Cohen Milstein suit against Golden Living continued. However, the core lawsuit against Golden Living was dismissed by Commonwealth Court on March 24, 2017. The case was pending appeal in the state Supreme Court at the time this book was published in late July 2018. Appendix C outlines the Commonwealth Court majority opinion and a dissenting justice's opinion. The entire majority opinion and the dissenting opinion are available to read on my website at https://www.wbeerman.com. The opinions cover, individually, 10 Golden Living objections to the AG's lawsuit.

Chapter 10: The Attorney General Lawsuits

On October 4, 2016, Kathleen Kane's successor, Pennsylvania Attorney General Bruce R. Beemer, announced a $2 million settlement with a different nursing home chain, Reliant Senior Care Holdings, which was discussed earlier. Cohen Milstein also participated in that suit.

Of the $2 million Reliant agreed to pay to the state, $1.25 million was to go to the Department of Health to improve regulatory oversight of nursing homes.

A Wilkes-Barre, PA *Times Leader* story about the settlement by Eileen Godin had a reader comment posted at the end by someone calling themselves Mickey Finn. It said: "And the mistreated patients and their families don't get squat."

When I asked about the participation of Cohen Milstein in the Reliant case and the distribution of the settlement proceeds, a spokesperson for the attorney general's office said:

"The Office of Attorney General did partner with Cohen Milstein on this (the Reliant) investigation. The firm has a tremendous amount of expertise in this field. Also, our use of outside counsel (Cohen Milstein) in this case allowed us to sort through a considerable volume of materials in a shorter time period. It would have been a huge undertaking for our staff attorneys working alone.

"In regard to the settlement, our office believes this was the appropriate way to resolve the case and ensure significant changes moving forward in the event Reliant operates these facilities in Pennsylvania (in the future)."

Chapter 10: The Attorney General Lawsuits

The attorney general's office provided me with court briefs and orders showing Cohen Milstein was paid $420,000, or 21 percent of the $2 million award, for work that it said included reviewing and summarizing 82,000 pages of documents, and performing 2,230 hours of investigation and litigation. The court approved the payment.

Regarding Cohen Milstein's participation in the New Mexico Preferred Care/Cathedral Rock case, AG attorney Juliet Keene told New Mexico First District Court Judge Sarah Singleton in open court on February 17, 2017:

"This case does not exist because of outside counsel (Cohen Milstein). This case exists because Cathedral Rock defrauded the State and caused a significant amount of unnecessary harm to elderly and disabled New Mexicans." Keene added: "It was just a matter of time . . . but these facilities that are the defendants in this case, they were on the pathway to prosecution by the Medicaid Fraud Control Unit for a very long time prior to Cohen Milstein. You know, outside counsel did not inform us about problems with these facilities, and now we are here." Continuing, Keene said her office received "hundreds and hundreds" of complaints between 1999 and 2014 about facilities that are defendants in the case.

I concluded that regardless of whether the defendants were guilty or not, the Kane-Beemer-Cohen Milstein Pennsylvania lawsuits and the New Mexico AG lawsuit had been among the more revealing sources of information that I found during my research. Also, even though nursing home residents did not get any money directly from the Reliant settlement, it seemed to me that in some cases the courts may be the last and best resort for alleged victims of abuse and neglect in nursing homes. Reliant admitted no

Chapter 10: The Attorney General Lawsuits

guilt in the settlement, the Golden Living suit was thrown out of Commonwealth Court, many nursing homes do provide good care, and many nursing home residents do not complain. Nevertheless, it seemed that in some cases lawyers and judges can be effective in overseeing nursing homes when government health oversight agencies are not.

I was concerned that Tom Price, a physician and former congressman who took over as secretary of health and human services on February 10, 2017, was an advocate of limiting the legal options available to aggrieved health care consumers. At one point, Price's Obamacare replacement bill reportedly would have created state administrative tribunals to hear cases of alleged malpractice, in lieu of jury trials.

In the 2015-2016 congressional election cycle, Price received $459,393 in campaign contributions from the health sector, among his total PAC money donations of $1,277,538, according to the CRP. Contributions to Price from the hospital/nursing home sector amounted to $36,750; $6,000 of that came from the American Health Care Association, an association of nursing home operators.

Overall, according to the CRP, PACs contributed $55,727,511 to federal election candidates in the 2015-2016 election cycle. Of that, $6,057,309 came from the hospital/nursing home sector, and $675,327 came from the American Health Care Association.

I hoped the health care sector contributions would not result in curtailment of litigation options available to persons injured in the health care industry.

Chapter 11: The Pennsylvania Office of the Auditor General; Now You See Them, Now You Don't

During my research about government oversight of nursing homes, I found that the Pennsylvania Department of the Auditor General had been a "now you see them – now you don't" participant with regard to nursing home oversight.

The auditor general's office played high-profile roles in the late 1990s and in 2015, but for the 14 years between 2000 and 2015, the office did no significant audit on the subject of nursing homes. The Pennsylvania secretary of health asked the auditor general to do an audit in July 2015, after Pennsylvania Attorney General Kathleen Kane, in collaboration with a private law firm from Washington, D.C., filed a much publicized lawsuit against a Pennsylvania nursing home chain on July 1, 2015. The lawsuit is discussed in Chapter 10.

In his introduction to his July 25, 2016 report on the 2015-16 audit, Auditor General Eugene DePasquale said

Chapter 11: The Pennsylvania Auditor General

that despite improvements resulting from the 1990s audits, "recent media reports have raised new concerns about DOH and its effectiveness in overseeing nursing homes and responding to complaints. In response to these criticisms, DOH requested that we conduct a performance audit to provide an independent assessment of DOH's mission with respect to nursing homes."

I thought this audit was a little late. On July 23, 2012, I wrote to former Pennsylvania Auditor General Jack Wagner, who served from January 18, 2005 until January 15, 2013, to suggest an audit about the "Effectiveness of Nursing Home Oversight." Subsequently, I discovered that nursing home oversight had been a hot topic in the news in Pennsylvania in the late 1990s.

In my 2012 email, I wrote:

"I recently filed a detailed complaint about a nursing home through the Pennsylvania Health Department's website. When I called a few days later to see if my complaint had arrived okay, I was astounded to find out the investigation had already been completed. Later, I received a letter in which the agency blew off about a half dozen of my complaints and confirmed one.

"As a retired certified internal auditor, I found the comments in the (health) department's reply letter to be amazingly contrary to logic. Equally amazing was a supervisor's explanation of the methodology used to investigate complaints. If an audit of the effectiveness of the state's nursing home oversight process is something you would be interested in, I would be happy to provide details supporting a conclusion that the oversight is not effective, is a waste of money, and fails to protect nursing home residents."

Chapter 11: The Pennsylvania Auditor General

I received a reply on July 24, 2012, from Stephanie G. Maurer, then deputy auditor general for performance audits. She wrote:

"Auditor General Jack Wagner has asked me to thank you for your email ... about your concerns regarding nursing home oversight by the Pennsylvania Department of Health.

"In March 1998, then-Auditor General Robert P. Casey Jr. [auditor general from 1997 to 2005], who is now a U.S. senator, released a performance audit about that very subject ("Residents in Jeopardy" was the title), followed by yet another audit ("Residents Still in Jeopardy"), and then a substantial amount of attention and additional work, including the formation of a task force.

"As I remember, there were significant changes, improvements, and communications that resulted from all that was done.

"Your suggestion that still more improvements are needed is one that I will keep on hand; I am also forwarding this email to the other audit deputy (Thomas Marks) and to the two bureau directors who conduct performance audits.

"Although our audit schedule is already determined for at least the remainder of the year, I am asking the recipients to keep your contact information on file for potential use during our next round of audit planning."

Maurer sent copies of her email to Marks, as well as to Helen Weigel, director of special performance audits, and to Janet Ciccocioppo, director of state and federal audits. However, Wagner left office as auditor general in January 2013.

Chapter 11: The Pennsylvania Auditor General

Regarding the past audits mentioned by Maurer, on March 11, 1998, former Auditor General Casey released the first of two performance audits that, according to a July 23, 1998 news release from Casey, found that the "Department of Health had failed miserably in its oversight of nursing home care." The news release referred to "Residents in Jeopardy" and "Residents Still in Jeopardy" as two "scathing" performance audits of the oversight of nursing home care in Pennsylvania.

I had moved out of Pennsylvania in 1978. Later, as a resident of New Mexico, and prior to that, Washington, D.C, and southern New Jersey, I was not aware of any state-level issues involving Pennsylvania nursing homes prior to my communication with Maurer after my mother's death.

Among the findings in the two Casey audits were one that Pennsylvania had not been aggressive in imposing sanctions against nursing homes. Statistics showed that in 1996, the Department of Health issued only 45 sanctions, 58 fewer than it issued in 1994, a year in which there were 41 fewer licensed facilities. (Amazingly, as noted earlier, in Chapter 9, the DOH took only two enforcement actions in 2012, so after some attention and improvement resulting from the Casey audits, the DOH apparently regressed, and one might comment, "Residents Still in Jeopardy – Again!")

One of the complaints highlighted in a Casey audit was about a nursing home patient suffering from dehydration, which struck a resonant chord with me because dehydration was also the subject of the lone health department citation in Mary Regina's case in 2011, 13 years after the Casey news release.

Chapter 11: The Pennsylvania Auditor General

In another finding especially interesting to me, the auditor general found "Pennsylvania families are not provided with sufficient information to select a nursing facility for their loved ones." Mary Regina and I had also become victims of that problem in 2011.

I attempted to follow up with Maurer in late November, 2015, but learned that she was no longer with the state auditor general's office.

I then wrote to Pennsylvania Auditor General Eugene DePasquale, who became auditor general on January 15, 2013, and searched the auditor general's website for audits about nursing homes or facilities. I found only one audit, about a nursing facility for a school district, and a follow-up audit report issued in 2000.

My email to DePasquale was replied to by John Murray, a regional director for administration, on December 2, 2015. He said the agency was "currently auditing the Department of Health" and agreed to forward information provided by me to the audit team.

The audit referred to by Murray was the one requested by State Secretary of Health Dr. Karen Murphy, PhD, in July 2015, shortly after the state attorney general filed the Golden Living lawsuit discussed in Chapter 10. As stated in Chapter 10, the essence of the Golden Living lawsuit was a claim that because staffing was inadequate in some nursing homes in the Golden Living chain, they could not deliver the services for which they were billing private customers and the State of Pennsylvania. Millions of dollars were at stake in the Golden lawsuit.

The DePasquale audit dovetailed with the argument by the plaintiffs in the Golden case. The audit report said:

Chapter 11: The Pennsylvania Auditor General

"Most in need of immediate improvement" was the audit finding that "residents' quality of life/care may be directly impacted by a nursing home's ability to provide direct nursing care .... Pennsylvania regulations governing nursing homes require that nursing homes provide at least 2.7 hours of direct nursing care, per resident, per day. We found that DOH lacked the requisite policies and procedures to guide its staff to ensure that nursing homes met this regulatory requirement."

The 81-page DePasquale audit report, which covered DOH operations during the period January 1, 2014 to October 31, 2015, also cited the DOH for deficiencies regarding handling of complaints and insufficient imposition of sanctions against poor-performing facilities.

"Before we began our work, a perfect storm was on the horizon because of inadequate review and enforcement," DePasquale said in a news release.

When auditors reviewed annual surveys (inspections) from 42 nursing homes, they found that 71 percent of the DOH staffing reviews were incomplete:

- 10 percent lacked any documentation showing that a review of the facility's staffing levels was conducted.
- In 37 percent of the surveys, DOH reviewed only 1 week of staffing information instead of the recommended 3 weeks.
- Of the 24 facility reviews that analyzed 3 weeks of staffing, only 50 percent also contained supporting documentation.

"What is worse," said the auditors, "is that DOH used inconsistent methods, such as averaging direct nursing care time over a week rather than determining daily care time, so facilities were not all held to the same standard."

"Then," added the auditors, "DOH did little to enforce the 2.7-hour law. Auditors found that, out of the 7,235 instances in which DOH completed a nursing home survey, it issued just 13 citations (for failure to meet the 2.7-hour standard) -- only 0.2 percent of the time."

"That is an unbelievably low number," DePasquale said. "Clearly, prior to this audit, DOH was not getting to the root of the problem, which likely is that some facilities may lack sufficient nursing staff.

"It's very simple: If nursing homes aren't sufficiently staffed, the quality of life and quality of care for residents will suffer," DePasquale said.

He noted that regulations allowed DOH to order increased facility staffing above the 2.7-hour standard, but DOH had never exercised that authority.

Criticizing the administration of former Republican Governor Tom Corbett, Jr. (January 18, 2011 to January 20, 2015), DePasquale, a Democrat, said:

"Responding to nursing home complaints should be one of DOH's most important responsibilities. Yet, for 3 years — beginning in July 2012 under the Corbett administration — DOH did not accept anonymous complaints. This was a direct violation of the federal Centers for Medicare & Medicaid Services' policy, which states that DOH must ensure the 'privacy and anonymity' of every person making a complaint.

"For 3 years, DOH risked nursing home residents' safety by ignoring anonymous complaints," DePasquale said.

Chapter 11: The Pennsylvania Auditor General

After DOH began accepting anonymous complaints in July 2015, the number of complaints increased by 63 percent, according to the audit report.

As noted in Chapter 9, 2012, 2013, and 2014, during the Corbett Administration, were the 3 years with the fewest enforcement actions during the period 2002-2015.

A July 26, 2016 Pennsylvania news headline by publisher PennLive on a story written by Daniel Simmons-Ritchie said: "Auditor General Slams Corbett-Era ban on Nursing Home Complaints." The story quoted DePasquale as saying "Getting rid of that (anonymous complaint process), in my view, was a decision intended to silence critics." Governor Corbett's comments are provided in Chapter 9.

Regarding sanctions, the audit report said that during the 22-month audit period, DOH cited 9,189 federal deficiencies in nursing homes and the federal government imposed more than $2 million in fines on Pennsylvania nursing homes. In contrast, DOH issued only 47 state sanctions, of which 32 were fines. The state fines totaled only $172,350, the auditors said.

DOH officials told the auditors they preferred to mandate training in response to deficiencies rather than levy fines. However, the auditors pointed out that during the 22 months covered by the audit, only 30 in-service training days were ordered for nursing homes.

The auditors said that although the state inspectors documented the reasons for sanctions, they did not document deficiencies that did not result in sanctions.

"DOH has considerable administrative discretion when pursuing sanctions, and we agree that not every instance of noncompliance may warrant a fine," DePasquale said.

"However, when a facility is not sanctioned but could have been, there needs to be an explanation."

As noted earlier, I believed DOH had not adequately explained or supported why it did not uphold most of my complaints and coded the one citation it did issue as "no actual harm."

Regarding the issue of down-coding the scope and severity codes for deficiencies cited by DOH, the auditors said they reviewed seven deficiencies rated severity/scope level code D or E, meaning "no actual harm," to determine whether the deficiencies may have warranted a higher severity rating. The auditors said DOH personnel convinced them the ratings were reasonably justified. However, these deficiencies all pertained to the limited category of pressure sores, a special emphasis area, and were not representative of the universe of scope and severity coding practices.

DePasquale credited Secretary Murphy with implementing corrective actions while the audit was still ongoing. Those actions are discussed in Chapter 9.

Responding to the audit report, the Pennsylvania Health Care Association (PHCA) said "any discussion of changes to the regulations also needs to include a frank discussion of the financial challenges fueled by chronic underfunding of nursing home care under the Medicaid program and the availability of a competent, highly skilled workforce."

The association, which represents more than 500 Pennsylvania long-term care and senior service providers, said:

Chapter 11: The Pennsylvania Auditor General

"More stringent penalties do not alone improve care. It is important to note that when any sanction or penalty is considered, the most important goal is to identify the practice in question, take steps to correct the practice, and ensure that any sanction does not jeopardize the facility's ability to improve resident care, comfort, and safety. Taking financial resources away from the bedside does not improve residential care."

PHCA and the Center for Assisted Living Management said in an August 2015 news release that the reimbursement rates under the Medicaid program fell $23 per day per resident short of the true cost of care.

According to PHCA, Pennsylvania's skilled nursing providers employed more than 120,000 women and men and provided care to approximately 80,000 residents every day.

The audit did not discuss the fact that in 2010, Title VI of the Patient Protection and Affordable Care Act (Obamacare) added a requirement that CMS establish a national automated system to collect and report payroll data on nurse staffing hours directly from nursing home payrolls. This requirement, still being implemented by CMS in 2016, presumably would help resolve staffing and staffing-review issues raised in the audit.

According to Government Accountability Office (GAO) report 16-33 of November 2015, CMS issued a memo outlining a plan to begin collecting staffing data through its payroll-based system on a voluntary basis beginning October 2015 and on a mandatory basis beginning July 2016 – the month the DePasquale audit report was issued. The goal is that the staffing-data

Chapter 11: The Pennsylvania Auditor General

collection system will be auditable to check the accuracy of the nursing home staffing data it contains.

However, a new set of CMS regulation revisions about nursing homes unveiled in 2016 did not include federal numerical minimum staffing requirements for nursing homes, such as the one calling for 2.7 hours of direct nursing care per day in Pennsylvania. So, although the staffing data collection system would compile staffing data, there was no national numerical federal standard with which to compare nursing home staffing levels. Nursing home resident advocacy groups wanted a 4.1-hour standard and expressed concern about CMS's failure to establish a federal numerical staffing standard.

Finally, in following up on recommendations from the 1990s audits, which included a recommendation that DOH develop a nursing home "report card," the DePasquale auditors said in 2016 that more could be done to help Pennsylvania citizens in their decision-making process as they select nursing homes. As noted, choosing the wrong nursing home had dreadful consequences for Mary Regina and me in 2011.

The auditors said that 29 items recommended for a nursing home report card are now published on the DOH website, but items such as nursing home owner, administrator, and management company are not readily apparent. The auditors also observed that staffing and quality measures – two key components of the CMS Five-Star system established in 2008, were self-reported by the nursing homes, "and as such, may not be reliable."

The auditors commented, "DOH has greatly improved the amount of information it presents on its website and now provides helpful information for consumers who may need a nursing home .... While these improvements are helpful, we believe DOH could better organize the data into meaningful rating categories, like a report card." The auditors said the report card should allow consumers to evaluate the performance of Pennsylvania-based nursing homes.

DOH said it was interested in pursuing the report card option, but it has been limited by budgetary constraints.

Chapter 12:
The Five-Star Rating System, and the U.S. Government Accountability Office's Audit

I looked into what Robert P. Casey, Jr. was doing about nursing homes since he transitioned from Pennsylvania auditor general to U.S. senator on the Senate Health, Education, Labor, and Pensions Committee.

In August 2015 Casey requested that the Government Accountability Office (GAO) audit the Five-Star rating system that the Centers for Medicare & Medicaid Services (CMS) uses to rate nursing homes and make the ratings public on the Medicare website, Medicare.gov (located under the heading: *Find a nursing home*).

GAO released a report on the results of its audit of the Five-Star system on December 6, 2016. The audit was critical of the Five-Star system, and echoed other critics who said the system failed to account for the experiences and opinions of nursing home residents regarding their nursing homes. Some of the results of the audit and other

Chapter 12: The Five-Star Rating System

evaluations of the Five-Star system are presented later in this chapter.

The Five-Star system is much more well known today than it was in 2011 when I chose Mary Regina's nursing home. For example, *U.S. News and World Report* bases its ratings of nursing homes partly on the CMS Five-Star system, although in 2016 *U.S. News* put caps on its own star ratings for nursing homes that have low ratings in medical quality measures.

Just as the health department is supposed to oversee nursing homes in Pennsylvania and the state auditor general and the inspector general can audit the health department's oversight effectiveness, nursing homes are overseen at the national level by CMS, and GAO and the Department of Health and Human Services inspector general can audit CMS.

CMS establishes regulations that nursing homes participating in Medicare and Medicaid are required to follow, as noted earlier. CMS designates an agency within each state to monitor nursing home compliance with CMS's regulations.

CMS established an initial version of the rating system in 2008 and periodically modifies it. CMS relies on state agencies such as the Pennsylvania Department of Health to conduct "surveys" (inspections) of nursing homes in the respective states and feed the resulting information in to CMS for oversight and use in the ratings. The nursing homes themselves also feed other rating data to CMS, following policy direction that CMS provides.

After learning of the then ongoing GAO audit of the Five-Star system in January 2016, I contacted GAO, offering to share my experience regarding my mother and inquiring how the audit was going. I called Dr. Linda T. Kohn, PhD, GAO's Director of Health Care Issues, and she referred me to Karin Wallestad, assistant director of the Health Care team. After conversing with Wallestad, I wrote the following letter.

William J. Beerman
3340 Squaw Mountain Drive
Las Cruces, NM 88011
Phone: 575-532-9398
Email: WilliamBeermanSr@Comcast.net

February 1, 2016

Ms. Karin Wallestad
U.S. Government Accountability Office
441 G. Street NW
Washington, DC 20548

Dear Ms. Wallestad,

Thank you for taking time to talk with me on January 29 about my experiences with my mother's nursing home and the Pennsylvania Department of Health (DOH), Division of Nursing Home Facilities, Bureau of Facility Licensure and Certification.

I will spare you the details of the complaint I filed with the Pennsylvania DOH and their reply.

Chapter 12: The Five-Star Rating System

However, I am attaching a summary of a few issues that I encountered which might be pertinent to your audit of the Five-Star Rating System, since nursing home complaint investigations logically would factor into ratings. I noticed that your 2015 audit, "CMS Should Continue to Improve Data and Oversight" (GAO-16-33), poses the question of why consumer complaints are up since 2005 while deficiencies identified in surveys are down. My limited personal experience leads me to think one reason probably is that the survey/investigation processes are constrained.

Also, I would like to say that my mother and my family suffered severely because we were not aware of the Five-Star Rating System and we could have benefitted profoundly from it had we known.

Sincerely,

//s//WILLIAM J. BEERMAN

Attachments:

(1) Summary of Issues
(2) Example of Hospital Attestation Report
(3) Internal Nursing Home Complaint that DOH Declined to Review

Chapter 12: The Five-Star Rating System

SUMMARY OF ISSUES

1. **The methods that the Pennsylvania Department of Health (DOH) used in 2012 to investigate complaints regarding my mother's nursing home were restricted and as a result the investigation was not completely effective. I wonder whether the investigative methods have changed?** Specifically, a DOH supervisor in Pittsburgh told me investigators were not allowed to consider any information other than what they found or heard during their 1-day onsite investigation at the nursing home. Relevant information such as reports from hospitals where patients had been sent from the nursing home were not considered. For example, findings on an intake report and an attestation report prepared by a hospital were not considered when the investigator dismissed all but one of my half-dozen well-documented complaints. Among hospital findings not considered was an attestation report entry documenting "Injury or poisoning occurring at/in residential institution [critical digoxin poisoning]." A sample attestation report is attached.

Also, the investigators declined to return to the nursing home to question a director of nursing who had been absent on the day that an investigator did the onsite investigation. The director of nursing had told me in a phone conversation that my written complaint to the nursing home about inappropriate administration of a controlled medication

Chapter 12: The Five-Star Rating System

(morphine) to my mother had been verified in an internal review by the nursing home, yet the DOH supervisor stuck to the DOH position that no medication error had occurred. The local supervisor would not even comment on whether the investigator had seen the formal written complaint document that I had submitted to the nursing home, which had a section for "Action to be Taken" by the nursing home. I suspect medications were administered by a nurse's aide who may not have been authorized to administer them, which caused harm. (See attached internal nursing home comment/complaint form.)

Also, the 1-day onsite investigation seemed to be rushed, and the priority seemed to be speed and the number of investigations that could be done in a given time period rather than the effectiveness of the investigations.

2. **Records of nursing homes were suspect**. A package of records delivered by the nursing home in response to my request for my mother's records did not include all pertinent documents. Further, one record apparently had been altered to show that a vital-signs temperature check ordered by a physician during an "infection watch" had been done. A photocopy of the same record that I happen to have showed the column for the check was blank. Apparently the check had not been done but the record later was changed to show it had been done. This is an example of why investigations should not rely solely on information provided by the nursing

home, especially if other sources are available.

3. **<u>Severity indicators may not be accurate</u>**. I found out 4 years after my mother's death that a DOH federal citation about failure of the nursing home to provide doctor-ordered IV hydration for my mother for at least 4 consecutive days, or 12 nursing shifts, resulted in a Code D severity classification. As best I can determine, Code D is part of Level II, which means "no more than minimal discomfort to the resident." At the time the code was assigned, DOH personnel knew my mother had died. The nursing home sent my mother to the hospital emergency room because of dehydration, sepsis, and other problems she had developed during her short stay at the nursing home. She never made it out of the hospital, and died there 10 days later. Even if she had not died, should an ambulance trip to an emergency room while unconscious and suffering from sepsis be considered "no more than minimal discomfort"? *<u>To what degree do such severity codings figure into the Five Star ratings?</u>* Because I was not made aware of how to find out and decipher the cryptic severity code, I did not have an opportunity to challenge the inappropriate coding at the time.

4. **<u>Public awareness of the Five-Star Rating System was insufficient.</u>** When asking my family to move my mother to a nursing/rehabilitation facility as soon as possible, the hospital that repaired her broken hip did not inform us that such facilities had government ratings. The hospital gave us a list of

Chapter 12: The Five-Star Rating System

nursing homes that showed no ratings. The hospital also told us the hospital staff were not allowed to recommend nursing homes. As a result, a somewhat frail patient who nevertheless would have had good prospects for recovery in a better nursing home was transferred to a below-average two-star nursing home although a four-star nursing home was located just 3 minutes, or 1 mile, away. I believe my inadvertent selection of a below-average nursing home was the root cause of my mother's demise. After learning of the ratings, the family visited the four-star facility 1 mile down the road twice and concluded that indeed there was a discernable difference in the quality levels of the two facilities. However, by then it was too late to move my mother, because she had developed a contagious infection requiring isolation at the two-star facility.

5. **Opinions of residents and their families about the results of investigations apparently are not tracked.** Comments on the investigation methods and results, and the severity code, should be solicited from patients and family members for the record. As of January 2016, the DOH solicited comments on a Complaint Quality Assurance Questionnaire. However, at the top of the questionnaire is the statement: "<u>N</u>ote: The purpose of this survey is not to assess the outcome of the investigation, but to ensure timely staff response and notification of the findings to the consumer." People with comments about the outcome of investigations, as opposed to the timeliness, are asked to contact the local DOH office supervisor.

However, such contacts with the local supervisor are likely to be made in phone calls, as in my case, and such oral information might never get captured in a survey, management records, databases, or ratings.

6. **<u>Below-average performance was repeated</u>**. I found that my mother's nursing home, rated two stars, below average, at the time of her death, was rated two stars when I checked 4 years later in 2016. I was unable to determine whether the rating had fluctuated during the 4 years, but I wondered how many residents over the years had suffered from the same below-average care as my mother had.

<u>Suggestions for CMS actions</u>.
- Establish procedures to ensure hospitals advise families that government ratings are available to assist them in selecting a nursing home.
- If the policy still exists, change the policy that limits investigator reviews to only records and information provided by, or learned at, the nursing home.
- To utilize millions of patients and their families as resources in nursing home oversight, encourage them to comment in the satisfaction survey process, and require nursing homes to provide the DOH hotline number and also a CMS hotline number to patients and their families. Then, if sufficient personnel resources are not available to properly investigate complaints, <u>shift resources from routine periodic surveys to complaint investigations</u>. This

Chapter 12: The Five-Star Rating System

would focus more attention in the nursing home oversight process on actual patient experiences and enable the DOH to spend more time and effort on more thorough and effective complaint investigations. Investigators drawn to nursing homes to investigate complaints naturally would also observe other nursing home practices while there.

- To enhance accuracy of severity codes and ratings, add additional procedures for cases in which a nursing home sends a resident to a hospital. A copy of the hospital intake report, showing the condition of the patient when they arrived at the hospital, and especially in the case of a fatality, the Attestation Report (e.g., Softmed Systems, Inc), should be incorporated into the nursing home record for review by investigators or obtained from the hospital by investigators who investigate a complaint. (See attached sample)
- Comments from patients and family about the outcome of investigations should be captured in writing and directed not only to the health department or other entity that did the investigation, but also to a third party such as CMS.

Chapter 12: The Five-Star Rating System

Western Pennsylvania Hospital - Forbes Regional Campus Page 1 of 2
Attestation Report

Patient Name: Beerman, Regina		Account #: 700031292621	Medical Record #: 2598414	
Admit Date 7/27/2011		Discharge Date 8/7/2011	LOS 11	
Age at Admit 86 years		Race White		
Attend Phys 011064 Muthappan, Palanlappan		Sex Female		
Date of Birth 6/1/1925		Financial Class M Medicare A & B		
Patient Type J Isolation Inpatient			Payor 1 M01 Medicare Part A	
Det Pt Type ID Inpt Discharged			Payor 2 C05 AARP	
Admit Dx 599.0 Urin. tract infection NOS			Payor 3	
Discharge Status DBZ, 20 Exp. at Med Fac. Autopsy Unknown				
Transfer Destination				

DRG		MDC	Weight	GMLOS	ALOS	Coder ID	Coded Date
871	SEPTICEMIA OR SEVERE SEPSIS W018		1.9074	5.40	7.20	MRCKK	8/15/2011

Seq.	Diagnosis		
1	038.3	Y	Septicemia due to anaerobes
2	348.30	Y	Encephalopathy, unspecified
3	518.81	N	Acute respiratory failure
4	486	Y	Pneumonia, organism unspecified
5	532.40	Y	Chronic/unspecified duodenal ulcer with hemorrhage, without mention of obstruction
6	008.45	Y	Intestinal infection due to Clostridium difficile
7	491.21	Y	Obstructive chronic bronchitis with (acute) exacerbation
8	285.1	Y	Acute posthemorrhagic anemia
9	995.91	Y	Sepsis
10	277.7	Y	Dysmetabolic syndrome X
11	294.8	Y	Persistent mental disorders due to conditions classified elsewhere
12	V10.05	E	Personal history of malignant neoplasm of large intestine
13	V10.3	E	Personal history of malignant neoplasm of breast
14	V15.88	E	Personal history of fall
15	V15.82	E	Personal history of tobacco use
16	416.8	Y	Chronic pulmonary heart disease
17	783.0	Y	Anorexia
18	427.31	Y	Atrial fibrillation
19	244.9	Y	Unspecified acquired hypothyroidism
20	V45.01	E	Status post cardiac pacemaker in situ
21	V45.82	E	Percutaneous transluminal coronary angioplasty status
22	414.00	Y	Coronary atherosclerosis of unspecified type of vessel, native or graft
23	972.1	Y	Poisoning by cardiotonic glycoside & drug of similar action
24	E858.3	Y	Accidental poisoning by agent affecting cardiovascular system
25	E849.7	Y	Injury or poisoning occurring at/in residential institution
26	V58.65	E	Long-term (current) use of steroids
27	782.3	Y	Edema
28	780.09	Y	Alteration of consciousness
29	428.0	Y	Congestive heart failure, unspecified
30	V58.61	E	Long-term (current) use of anticoagulants

			AN	FC	AT
Dictation	H&P	Consults:			
Confirmation	OR	Consults:			
Number	D/C	Consults:			

Above is an Attestation Report showing, for example, Line Item 25, *Injury or poisoning occurring at/in residential institution.*

Chapter 12: The Five-Star Rating System

COMPLAINT I FILED
WITH MRNH RESIDENT COMMENT FORM
(AS AN ATTACHMENT)

JULY 26, 2011

On a number of occasions members of my family and I have found my mother to be in a head-dangling, apparently drug-induced stupor for entire days.

Most recently this happened on Sunday and Monday, July 24 and 25.

Notably, I found my mother this way the morning of the 25th, when I came in about 8 a.m. anticipating my taking her to the doctor at 10 a.m. I was told she had had a panic attack and had been given morphine and Klonapin at 6 a.m. -- even though she was on the antidepressant Paxil. She remained virtually non-rousable throughout the day, and went to the doctor in an ambulance with her mouth agape the entire trip. I'm sure she didn't even know she had been to the doctor. Upon seeing her, the doctor expressed surprise, saying that the last time he had seen her she was alert.

I was concerned about what was causing these anxiety attacks – what was my mother so afraid of? So I decided to come in early on the 26th and possibly witness one and hear what she was saying, or at least ask her nurse what my mother had said she was anxious about.

When I arrived at about 5:45 a.m., I asked her nurse at that time how my mother was doing. The nurse, ▮▮▮▮, said she had very low consciousness (I forget the exact

Chapter 12: The Five-Star Rating System

words) and that the nurse had delayed giving her meds because she was afraid she might choke. The nurse said my mother had been out all night. This means that my mother had been in the stupor for 24 hours.

I determined that my mother's nurse the mornings of the 24th and 25th had been ████████, who happened to be working downstairs this morning. I went downstairs to ask ███ what my mother had been so anxious about.

███ said my mother "didn't say anything." I asked if she said she was in pain and ███ said no. ███ said my mother had been coughing. She said she gave the morphine because my mother was moaning.

Then I asked about the previous morning (Sunday) and she said "It wasn't like a full-flown panic attack. Like she wasn't hyperventilating like some patients do. Nothing like that."

I wonder if this drugging of my mother was necessary? Does the facility have controls and procedures to monitor/guide the administration of strong drugs by non-doctors?

We had expressed concern before about over-medication. At our suggestion the doctor had reduced her morphine dosage to .5 mg, and we thought the practice of giving morphine and Klonapin together had been stopped.

These stupors have consequences. First it cannot be good for a patient to lie motionless around the clock. When I last saw her on the 25th she was asleep in her bed with her head askew with her bed control and her alert button on the floor. Does it affect circulation and respiration to lie motionless for days? My mother is supposed to be turned and moved every 2 hours. In the last 2 days she has missed six meals, and already had an eating problem and was on an appetite enhancer. Also, the therapist wrote on her therapy ortho update July 25, "Unable to arouse for therapy [due to] meds."

I forwarded a copy of my letter to GAO on to CMS. The CMS reply is presented later in this chapter.

* * *

Academic Study

The Five-Star Rating System on the Nursing Home Compare (NHC) website has been criticized for not reflecting the opinions of nursing home residents and their families about the nursing homes rated.

As noted earlier, I suggested to GAO, CMS, and the Pennsylvania Department of Health that feedback from residents and family members about nursing homes and the results of complaint investigations be captured and utilized in nursing home oversight.

A 2014 report published by the Gerontological Society of America recommended that the Five-Star system be refined to include a consumer component. The report, written by Anthony Williams, master of gerontological studies, MBA, Jane K. Straker, PhD, and Robert Applebaum, PhD, concluded that the existing rating system did not adequately reflect the satisfaction of consumers – residents of nursing homes and their families.

The report noted that three of the four Five-Star ratings categories were based on data related to staffing, performance measured against quality indicators, and information from health inspections. The fourth category, the overall rating, was derived from the first three. But

Chapter 12: The Five-Star Rating System

there was no component measuring consumer satisfaction in the ratings.

The study analyzed the relationship between star ratings and data about nursing home satisfaction collected from Ohio nursing home residents and their families. Ohio was one of six states that publicly reported consumer satisfaction data.

After analyzing detailed comparisons between individual nursing home star ratings in each of the four rating categories (staffing, quality measures, inspections, and overall rating), and consumer satisfaction data, the report authors said there were significant inconsistencies between some of the ratings and the consumer satisfaction data.

Many nursing homes that received five stars on the NHC overall rating had moderate to very low levels of consumer satisfaction, and many nursing homes that received one star on the NHC overall rating had high to very high consumer satisfaction. With high rates of inconsistency between NHC overall ratings and consumer satisfaction scores, it is difficult to say that consumer views of nursing homes are adequately reflected in the NHC overall rating, the authors said.

The report also said that because of the levels of inconsistency with consumer satisfaction levels in the various ratings categories, "...inferring how satisfied customers might be with nursing homes based on NHC star ratings is not viable."

The report concluded:

"At a minimum, the complete exclusion of consumer satisfaction data from NHC is cause for concern. In order to serve as a more comprehensive and reliable resource for customers, CMS could work to better integrate the thoughts and opinions of consumers into its NHC star rating system .... Although incorporating resident satisfaction into the star rating system presents some challenges, [report] data indicate that the failure to include consumers is a serious limitation in the current star rating system."

Center for Medicare Advocacy Article

An article entitled, "Don't Be Fooled by the Federal Nursing Home Five-Star Quality Rating System," was published by Toby Edelman, a senior policy attorney for the Center for Medicare Advocacy, on October 5, 2016.

The article said that in a research sample, self-reporting by nursing homes in two of the star subcategories generally boosted the overall composite rating by one star level – for example, from a one-star overall rating to a two-star overall rating, or from a four-star overall rating to a five-star overall rating.

Part of the study looked at data about Special Focus Facilities (SFF), which are nursing homes on a CMS watch list of poorly performing facilities. Higher scores in self-reported staffing and/or quality measures boosted nearly half of SFFs from their otherwise one-star overall composite rating to two-stars, the article said.

The research report referred to an August 24, 2014 *New York Times* article by Katie Thomas on the same subject entitled, "Medicare Star Ratings Allow Nursing Homes to Game the System." After doing its own research 2 years later, the Center for Medicare Advocacy concluded: "The Center's analysis indicates that data manipulation continues and ... this manipulation is likely influencing admission decisions."

The Edelman article also reported that "Five-star facilities also use their (self-reported) staffing and quality measure domains to boost their overall ratings to five stars." The article said this occurred in 96 percent of ratings for 113 skilled nursing facilities that had five stars as their overall rating for all 7 years since the Five Star Quality Rating System was introduced in December 2008.

The article concluded: "Providing composite scores is intended to help consumers make sense of the large amounts of material on *Nursing Home Compare*, but composite scores do a disservice to the public when nursing facilities' self-reported information boosts facilities' ratings to higher levels."

Pennsylvania Survey

A 2016 Pennsylvania Nursing Home Quality Improvement Task Force focus-group-type survey of residents of six nursing homes compared CMS's star ratings with the residents' own ratings. The survey is discussed in Chapter 14.

The residents participating in the survey ranked two nursing homes -- one a five-star and one a one-star -- the same as CMS. They ranked two other nursing homes higher than CMS by an average of 1.8 stars, and two nursing homes lower than CMS by an average of 0.9 stars.

Ratings Flip-flop

A 2016 report by the Pennsylvania Nursing Home Quality Improvement Task Force pointed out that between

Chapter 12: The Five-Star Rating System

2009 and 2013 the percentage of Pennsylvania nursing homes with one star was cut in half from 26 percent to 13 percent, and the percentage of Pennsylvania homes with five stars doubled from 12 percent to 23 percent, based on CMS data. The percentages in the middle, from two stars to four, remained essentially unchanged. The flip flop in the numbers for one- and five-star homes was similar in national statistics. The data was from a June 6, 2014 CMS report, "*Nursing Home Compare Five-Star Quality Rating System: Year Five Report.*"

I found it interesting that the numbers for two large Pennsylvania nursing home chains discussed in Chapter 6 reflected notably different distributions of star ratings in 2016 when I counted them. One chain had 14 percent of its nursing homes rated at five stars and 17 percent rated at one star. The other had 6 percent at five stars and 28 percent at one star.

GAO Audit

The GAO audit report on the Five-Star System, requested by three Democrats, Senator Casey, Senate Finance Committee ranking member Senator Ron Wyden, and Representative Elijah E. Cummings, the ranking member of the House Committee on Oversight and Government Reform, said that unless CMS makes enhancements to the Five-Star system, it cannot ensure the system fully meets its primary goal.

The report, dated November 2016 although it was not released to the public until December 6, is titled "NURSING HOMES: Consumers Could Benefit from Improvements to the Nursing Home Compare Website and Five-Star Quality Rating System (GAO-17-61)."

Chapter 12: The Five-Star Rating System

According to CMS, the primary goal of the Five-Star system is to provide consumers with an easy way to understand nursing home quality and distinguish between high- and low-performing nursing homes. A secondary goal of the system is to help improve nursing home quality by publicly reporting quality-of-care-information, which may provide an incentive for providers to improve their quality of care.

GAO said:

"Because the Five-Star system contains multiple types of information, compiled from different sources, and has complexities inherent in its rating systems, it can be challenging for consumers to fully understand how to take advantage of the varied information it contains.

"Additional capability and information not currently included in the rating system could also benefit consumers trying to differentiate between high- and low-performing nursing homes – such as the ability to compare homes nationally [not just within states] and the addition of consumer satisfaction survey information."

The auditors recommended that CMS:

- add information to the Five-Star system that allows consumers to compare nursing homes nationally;
- evaluate the feasibility of adding consumer satisfaction information to the Five Star system;
- and add certain explanatory and introductory information to the Five-Star website.

As a former editor of audit reports, I noticed that the recommendation about adding consumer satisfaction information was exceptionally weak for an audit recommendation, and I assumed the word choice was deliberate. I thought the recommendation should have said flatly, "Add consumer satisfaction information..." instead of merely "**Evaluate the feasibility of** adding consumer satisfaction information."

I noted that within the 42-page audit report, CMS contended that collecting consumer satisfaction information in a consistent, objective way was a challenge, but GAO pointed out that CMS had been able to add consumer satisfaction information to its separate rating system for hospitals. "Until consumer satisfaction information is included in the ratings system, consumers will continue to make nursing home decisions without the benefit of a key performance measure and may not be choosing the home that would best meet their needs," GAO said.

CMS disagreed with GAO's recommendation that it add information that would allow consumers to compare nursing homes nationally, across state borders. CMS said that because states' execution of standard nursing home surveys varies, it is difficult to compare survey results from state to state. However, GAO responded with a seemingly sharp retort that "efforts should have been and should continue to be made to reduce state variation in standard surveys."

In a joint news release on December 6, 2016, the congressional requestors of the audit commented on it. Senator Casey, noting that his home state of Pennsylvania has the fifth largest population of older citizens in the country, said, "This report makes important recommendations on how to improve this rating system. I call on CMS to move swiftly to implement these changes."

Chapter 12: The Five-Star Rating System

Senator Wyden said, "Selecting a nursing home is a consequential and challenging decision for seniors and their families, and they need the best information possible."

Representative Cummings said: "American families rely on CMS to publish meaningful ratings that will help guide them through difficult decisions they face when they seek nursing care for their family members. I encourage CMS to carefully consider these recommendations to ensure that the ratings accurately and clearly reflect the measures of comfort and quality that Americans expect from such a rating system."

*　*　*

On March 2, 2016, I forwarded my February 1, 2016 letter to GAO's Karin Wallestad on to Thomas Hamilton, director of CMS's Center for Clinical Standards and Quality/Survey and Certification Group. I asked whether conditions outlined in the letter still existed with regard to the complaint investigation process and the Five-Star rating system.

On May 23, 2016 I received a two-page, single spaced reply from David R. Wright, acting director, who had replaced Hamilton.

Responding to issues I raised regarding restricted survey methodology, need for review of records beyond the nursing home, and questionable severity codes for citations, Wright pointed out that CMS's State Operations Manual (SOM) is provided to all nursing home surveyors. It includes the regulations and guidance for investigating and applying the regulations. He explained that CMS provides ongoing surveyor training and guidance to state agencies to assist with the process of determining if a citation is present

Chapter 12: The Five-Star Rating System

and how to assign the appropriate scope and severity to that citation.

"The complaint survey process is a critical component of nursing home oversight," Wright said. However, he pointed out that according to the SOM, "the timing, scope, duration, and conduct of a complaint investigation are at the discretion of the State Agency, except when a determination is made that immediate jeopardy may be present or ongoing or a higher level of actual harm may be present.

"During the investigation, surveyors are directed to gather all pertinent information through observation, interviews of staff and residents and record reviews."

The SOM states that the surveyor will determine what sources of evidence are required to evaluate the non-compliance.

Wright commented, "Your letter asked if investigative methods have changed since 2012? While we have made changes to certain areas of the State Operations Manual, we have not changed our guidance relevant to the concerns you raised."

A check during 2016 showed Section 5300 of the SOM, "Investigation of Complaints for Nursing Homes," was last updated on March 17, 2006.

"While regulation precludes us from re-opening the 2012 survey of your mother's nursing home, we are sharing your specific concerns about that survey with the Philadelphia Regional Office," Wright said. "That office monitors and is responsible for performance oversight of the Pennsylvania Department of Health (DOH). We are requesting that your concerns be shared with DOH and

Chapter 12: The Five-Star Rating System

addressed through our ongoing performance management reviews of the state's operations."

Wright said, "We also appreciate your suggestion that an additional source of information would be gathering feedback from residents and their families following the complaint regarding both the process and timeliness of the investigation."

Chapter 13: At National and State Levels, Consumer Complaints Rise While Citations And Enforcement Actions Decline

Statistical evidence compiled and reported by the Government Accountability Office (GAO) shows the number of complaints about nursing homes rose while the number of serious deficiencies cited by nursing home oversight agencies declined. Similarly, data collected by the Centers for Medicare & Medicaid Services (CMS) showed a decline in enforcement actions.

Based on my own unscientific sample of one (my experience with my own complaint about my mother's nursing home), I am pretty sure the decrease in citations is a problem. I admit I may be somewhat biased on this point because of my first-hand observations, but I believe the root cause of the decrease in citations most likely is faulty government oversight of nursing homes.

Chapter 13: Complaints Up; Enforcement Down

As a former certified internal auditor, I know that fundamental principles of statistical sampling disallow drawing conclusions about the entire universe of nursing home complaints and citations from the results of my own personal sample of one case study about my mother's ordeal.

But common sense tells me that if the Pennsylvania Department of Health (DOH) blew off most of the issues in my well-documented complaint, and understated the severity code of the one violation they could not ignore, DOH might be acting similarly in other cases. And while the Pennsylvania DOH was not reporting or was downgrading deficiencies, other oversight agencies in other states might be doing the same thing.

The Pennsylvania DOH graded its citation regarding my mother as "Code D: No Actual Harm with Potential for More than Minimal Harm that Is Not Immediate Jeopardy." In short, this would commonly be referred to as a "No Actual Harm" deficiency. Following is a somewhat ambiguous Scope and Severity Grid for Rating Nursing Home Deficiencies from the 2015 CMS Nursing Home Data Compendium. The same chart appeared in the 2013 Compendium, which included deficiencies from 2011, when Mary Regina was going through her ordeal, and 2012, when my complaint was investigated. Some critics have questioned why "actual harm" is not considered more serious than "immediate jeopardy" in the chart.

The 2016 Nursing Home Data Compendium, with 2015 data, was not yet released as of June 2017.

Chapter 13: Complaints Up; Enforcement Down

	Isolated	Pattern	Widespread
Immediate Jeopardy in Resident Health or Safety	**J**	**K**	**L**
Actual Harm that is Not Immediate Jeopardy	**G**	**H**	**I**
No Actual Harm with Potential for More than Minimal Harm that is Not Immediate Jeopardy	**D**	**E**	**F**
No Actual Harm with Potential for Minimal Harm	**A**	**B**	**C**

Of course, I considered the "No Actual Harm" coding outrageous for the citation in my mother's case, in which she became unresponsive, had to be sent to the emergency room, had to have the ambulance diverted to a closer hospital during the trip, and, ultimately, died in the hospital.

I see my mother's story as flesh on the statistical skeleton that I believe depicts somewhat realistically the unsatisfactory state of some aspects of the government's oversight of nursing homes.

On November 30, 2015, GAO published a report to Congress that provided an intriguing context for me to ponder as I mulled over the ineffectiveness of the Pennsylvania DOH's investigation of my complaint about MRNH's treatment of my mother. The investigation is covered in Chapter 9.

The GAO Report (GAO-16-33) is entitled, *NURSING HOME QUALITY; CMS Should Continue to Improve Data and Oversight*.

GAO reported after a rigorous study that while citations issued by nursing home oversight agencies for serious deficiencies went down, consumer complaints about nursing homes went up.

As briefly mentioned earlier, CMS, an agency within the U.S. Department of Health and Human Services, defines the quality standards that nursing homes must meet in order to participate in the Medicare and Medicaid programs. To monitor compliance with these standards, CMS enters into agreements with agencies in each state's government to conduct required "surveys," or evaluations of the state's nursing homes, and to investigate complaints. In Pennsylvania, the DOH, which investigated my complaint about MRNH, is the designated state nursing home survey agency for CMS.

To identify trends in the number of consumer complaints regarding resident care or safety reported by residents, families, ombudsmen, or others, GAO analyzed data from CMS's Automated Survey Processing Environment/ Incident Tracking System (ASPE/ITS). Specifically, GAO calculated the total number of complaints reported (GAO emphasized that "reported" doesn't mean "substantiated") for all nursing homes for years 2005 through 2014.

Chapter 13: Complaints Up; Enforcement Down

To identify trends in the number of "serious" deficiencies (deficiencies at the actual harm or immediate jeopardy levels, alphabetical codes G through L) cited during nursing home standard surveys, GAO analyzed data from CMS's Certification and Survey Provider Enhanced Reports System for the years 2005 through 2014. Specifically, GAO calculated the number of serious deficiencies reported during standard surveys in each year.

Overall, GAO looked at four data sets. Three of them, (1) serious deficiencies cited on standard surveys, (2) staffing, and (3) selected clinical quality measures, showed movement in up or down directions that demonstrated "potential" quality improvements in nursing homes. As noted, deficiencies were reported by state survey agencies, such as the Pennsylvania DOH, but staffing and clinical quality measures were self-reported by the nursing homes themselves. The fourth data set, consumer complaints, which I considered to be the collective voice of dissatisfied residents, their families, and advocates, came from a CMS database (ASPE/ITS). The complaints data set showed an increase and therefore demonstrated a "potential" decrease in nursing home quality.

The citation in Mary Regina's case, coded "D," would not have been included in the GAO study because the deficiency did not meet the criteria of a serious deficiency. This caused me to doubt somewhat the usefulness of the CMS data, because downgrading of deficiencies such as the one pertaining to Mary Regina might be widespread.

From 2005 through 2014, according to GAO, the average number of consumer complaints that were reported increased nationally from 3.2 to 3.9 per nursing home, a 21 percent increase over the 10-year period. After an initial increase, the number of complaints decreased from 2008

Chapter 13: Complaints Up; Enforcement Down

through 2011, but then increased again from 2011 through 2014. (Pennsylvania, for example, had a reported average number of consumer complaints per nursing home of 2.4 in 2014, but for some undetermined reason none were recorded in the CMS database for 2005, so no comparison was possible.)

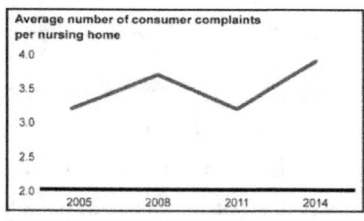 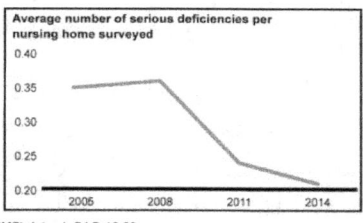

Source: GAO analysis of Centers for Medicare & Medicaid Services (CMS) data. | GAO-16-33

Specifically, GAO said 52,411 complaints were reported nationally in 2005, and 61,466 were reported in 2014.

Regarding deficiencies cited on standard surveys by state survey agencies such as the Pennsylvania DOH, GAO said that from 2005 through 2014, the number of serious deficiencies cited per nursing home surveyed decreased nationally from 0.35 to 0.21, a 41 percent decline over the 10 years. Specifically, 4,840 serious deficiencies were cited during surveys for 13,800 nursing homes in 2005, and 2,660 serious deficiencies were cited during surveys for 12,759 nursing homes for 2014. (In Pennsylvania, for example, the average number of serious deficiencies per home cited on standard surveys went from 0.22 in 2005 to 0.14 for 2014, a 35.7 percent decline.)

CMS stated in its March 25, 2016, Nursing Home Data Compendium, 2015 edition, that Level D "no actual harm" severity was the level assigned to 55.2 percent of deficiencies cited nationally in 2014. For contrast, the rating of Level G, "Actual Harm that is Not Immediate

Chapter 13: Complaints Up; Enforcement Down

Jeopardy," was assigned to only 2 percent of the deficiencies cited. Only 0.3 percent of deficiencies were characterized as Level J, "Immediate Jeopardy to Resident Health or Safety," the worst rating for individual deficiencies other than those that are part of a pattern (Level K) or are widespread (Level L).

In a March 26, 2016 memo to state survey agency directors about the 2015 Nursing Home Data Compendium, Thomas E. Hamilton, then director of the CMS Survey and Certifications Group, commented that "the percentage of surveys cited on standard nursing home deficiencies at scope and severity 'D' or 'E' reached 83.8% of all deficiencies in 2014, an unprecedented proportion." Both of these codes indicate "No Actual Harm." I emailed Hamilton to ask him what he thought was the reason for the "unprecedented" statistic and why it was noteworthy. Hamilton did not reply.

Subsequently, CMS pointed to "The Great Recession" as a reason for an overall decline in citations and enforcement actions, which is discussed later in this chapter.

GAO noted in its report (GAO-16-33): "Policymakers and others have questions about whether changes in reported nursing home quality represent actual improvements in quality or, for example, may be the result of changes in how oversight is performed." GAO said the congressional requestors of the audit "asked us to provide information on the quality of care in nursing homes and to study whether changes in quality are due to improvements in quality or to changes in oversight."

The American Health Care Association, which represents thousands of nursing homes, contends the

Chapter 13: Complaints Up; Enforcement Down

decline in deficiencies cited is evidence of improvement in the quality of nursing home care. The association's position is discussed later.

GAO said CMS's ability to assess nursing home quality trends is complicated by various issues regarding the data. It listed the following issues concerning data: state variations regarding recording of complaints; multiple survey types and state "challenges" in completing surveys that affect deficiencies cited on standard surveys; and self-reporting by nursing homes regarding selected quality measures and nurse staffing levels.

An example of an issue regarding citation of serious deficiencies was that some officials believed an automated electronic survey process that was being implemented resulted in fewer deficiencies being cited compared to the old paper process. In addition, in some cases, lack of a sufficient number of experienced surveyors, and surveyors being overworked, pushed down the number of deficiencies reported. An example of an issue regarding complaints was that implementation of a standardized complaint form made available on websites facilitated the filing of complaints.

On the other hand, as discussed in Chapter 11, the Pennsylvania auditor general said a 3-year suspension of acceptance of anonymous complaints materially suppressed the total number of complaints recorded in Pennsylvania.

GAO said that insufficient monitoring of the effects of changes in procedures also impaired the ability to evaluate nursing home quality.

The GAO report contained five pages about possible factors affecting the ability to assess quality trends.

Chapter 13: Complaints Up; Enforcement Down

However, I drew my own conclusions based on my own unscientific sample of one: the handling of my own complaint, which actually covered a half dozen different issues and could have been counted as six complaints. It occurred to me that whatever the cause for the increase in complaints, the complaints nevertheless were real complaints filed by real people. I thought it was very unlikely that a substantial increase in complaints should not be accompanied by an increase in citations. I thought that the illogical relationship between rising complaint numbers and declining citation numbers most likely was attributable to ineffectiveness in the oversight process.

Data released in CMS reports about nursing homes lagged substantially behind report issue dates. CMS released on March 25, 2016 the 2015 Nursing Home Data Compendium, which contained data from 5 years of nursing home survey outcomes through 2014 for more than 15,000 nursing homes participating in Medicaid and Medicare, and 4 years of data on the average of 1.4 million residents who resided in nursing homes each day. It did not contain explicit information about complaint investigation results. The 2016 compendium due out in 2017 would contain data from 2015. The 2016 compendium was overdue as this book was published in June 2017.

I could find no current national information about the results of investigations of actual complaints filed with state survey agencies, such as how many were considered worthy of investigations, how many were upheld, how many resulted in citations, and what severity codes were assigned. As noted, the citation information reported earlier in this chapter was about citations resulting from routine surveys, not complaint investigations.

Chapter 13: Complaints Up; Enforcement Down

Complaints specifically were addressed in a GAO audit, *More Reliable Data and Consistent Guidance Would Improve CMS Oversight of State Complaint Investigations* (GAO-11-280, April 7, 2011).

The report said: "Complaint investigations offer a unique opportunity to identify and correct potential care problems. They can provide more timely alerts of potential problems than standard surveys and target specific areas identified by residents, their families, nursing home staff, and others. In 2009, half of all violations of federal requirements that resulted in some level of harm to nursing home residents were cited during complaint investigations."

The 2011 report stated that among investigated complaints, 19 percent were substantiated and resulted in the citation of at least one federal deficiency.

Although GAO discussed various factors that possibly were contributing to a decrease in citations, CMS pointed to "The Great Recession" as a major factor. On June 3, 2016, CMS announced the posting online of data on nursing home enforcement actions. David R. Wright, director of the CMS Survey and Certification Group, sent to state survey agency directors a memo about the posting entitled "Enforcement Reports in Context: The Impact of the Recession."

The memo provided a chart showing the average number of deficiencies cited per survey, covering the years 1996-2014. The chart showed a general increase in citations per year from 1996 to 2006, followed by a downward trend from 2007 through 2014. The following graph is an excerpt from the CMS chart.

Chapter 13: Complaints Up; Enforcement Down

The change in average deficiencies cited per survey from 7.2 to 5.7 is a 21-percent decline.

Wright's June 3, 2016 memo states:

"This report provides data about enforcement actions taken during the years that state governments were experiencing budget constraints as a consequence of the Recession that began in December 2007. This recession is commonly referred to as the 'Great Recession' because the economic damage done to the economies of the United States and nations around the world was of historic proportions. To fully appreciate the enforcement data contained in this report, it is helpful to evaluate the survey and enforcement activities both before and after the Recession. The period before the Recession was notable for an increase in survey activities, initiatives, and deficiency citations, while the period after the Recession began is notable for a decline in overall survey activities and enforcement actions."

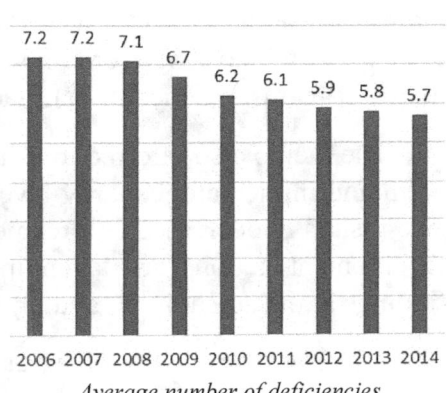

Average number of deficiencies cited per survey

The memo added:

"The Recession that began December 2007 officially lasted until June 2009, but its effects on state budgets and the economy in general lasted many years after the Recession ended. Most, if not all, State Survey Agencies were negatively impacted by the Recession. This led to widespread reports of layoffs, furloughs, hiring freezes, and

Chapter 13: Complaints Up; Enforcement Down

other measures that limited State Survey Agency oversight capacity. The Recession-based constraints affecting State Survey Agencies correlate with lower deficiency citation rates for the post-2009 period .... Lower deficiency citation rates inexorably lead to fewer opportunities for enforcement and therefore fewer enforcement actions imposed against a noncompliant facility."

The memo also referred to a "notable" decline in actual harm and immediate jeopardy level citations. "This decline also results in decreased enforcement activity because most enforcement actions are taken in response to deficiency findings at the actual harm and immediate jeopardy levels."

The CMS correlation of fewer deficiency citations with the Recession demonstrated to me that fewer citations actually did reflect a decline in oversight. Wright's memo did not attribute the decline in cited deficiencies to an increase in nursing home quality.

It occurred to me that if the Recession and/or other factors had caused a weakening of oversight and enforcement in nursing homes, there was little reason to assume conditions in nursing homes had improved since 2008. Such an assumption would be inconsistent with the increase in complaints. The Recession may have caused nursing homes to cut spending on staffing and other resources. Despite the decrease in citations, which some contend indicated an improvement in care, the increase in complaints most likely indicated that conditions actually got worse.

Asked about the impact of the Recession on Pennsylvania DOH oversight of nursing homes, a spokesperson for the secretary of health said in 2016, "The Department is not able to effectively comment on the

Chapter 13: Complaints Up; Enforcement Down

impact of the Recession on nursing home regulatory activity."

As noted, data in CMS reports and audits tended to be substantially older than the report publication dates.

A February 2014 report by the inspector general for the Department of Health and Human Services (HHS) contained 2011 data about harm that residents suffered in skilled nursing facilities. The report, OEI-06-11-00370, is entitled, "Adverse Events in Skilled Nursing facilities: National Incidence Among Medicare Beneficiaries."

If, because of the Recession or other factors, complaints have increased, and possibly conditions have not improved, the 2011 data might still be indicative of current conditions.

The report estimated that 22 percent of Medicare beneficiaries in skilled nursing facilities experienced adverse events during stays of 35 days or less

Adverse events were described in the HHS IG report as events that caused harm that fell into one of four categories: (1) the event prolonged the resident's nursing home stay, or required transfer to a hospital; (2) it contributed to or resulted in "permanent" harm; (3) it required intervention to sustain the resident's life, or (4) it contributed to or resulted in the resident's death. Most of the events fell into category 1 (79 percent); category 4 accounted for 6 percent.

In my assessment, my mother's 2011 case qualified for all four of the categories of "adverse event." But I doubt her case made it into the statistics.

The IG estimated that for residents who experienced adverse events in skilled nursing facilities that required

Chapter 13: Complaints Up; Enforcement Down

them to go to a hospital, the cost to Medicare was $2.8 billion in 2011. For my mother's post-nursing-home hospital stay, Medicare was billed for more than $10,000.

In addition to the events defined as "adverse," another 11 percent of residents experienced lesser, temporary harm, according to the IG.

***

At the risk of seeming politically biased, I could not help but notice that the period of declining enforcement actions discussed in Wright's memo, 2008-2014, and depicted in the preceding chart, not only was partly concurrent with the years after the Great Recession. It also was largely concurrent with the Obama administration, which began in 2008, and the implementation of the Affordable Care Act, which was passed in 2010. The Act contained provisions intended to strengthen oversight and enforcement penalties, expand staff training, and increase information on nursing home quality available to consumers and regulators.

In 2010, Title VI of the Affordable Care Act added a requirement that CMS establish a national system to collect electronically and report payroll data on direct care staffing levels, including nursing hours, turnover, and retention rates. This requirement was still being implemented by CMS in 2016.

I did not attempt to research the influence of the Act on the state of nursing home care.

Meanwhile, a nursing home industry lobbying group contended declines in nursing home citations were evidence of improvement in the quality of nursing home care.

Chapter 13: Complaints Up; Enforcement Down

In a news release on March 30, 2016, the American Health Care Association (AHCA), a federation of nursing home operators, commented on a tangential issue, the creation of regional elder justice task forces by the Department of Justice, but referred to a perceived decline in deficiencies in nursing homes:

Washington, D.C. *— AHCA President and CEO Mark Parkinson [who is a former governor of Kansas] made the following statement today about the Department of Justice's announcement of the 10 Regional Elder Justice Task Forces:*

*"America's skilled nursing care centers are united and focused on improving the quality of care we provide. Efforts like our national Quality Initiative push our profession forward and culminate in a culture of excellence. The results of these efforts speak for themselves. Data released just today by the Centers for Medicare & Medicaid Services shows that **deficiencies are down, demonstrating that quality is on the rise**.*

"We support any effort to improve overall care and weed out bad actors, but today's announcement [about the Elder Justice Task Forces] mistakenly conveys that quality is on the decline. It is a smokescreen aimed at finding cost cutting measures that would threaten life-improving post-acute and long-term care services for millions of seniors.

"Creating task forces under the guise of fraud and abuse is actually pointing a finger at a flawed Medicare payment system. We support comprehensive payment reforms, which would revolutionize the system to further enhance services while producing cost savings for the federal government."

Chapter 13: Complaints Up; Enforcement Down

According to its website, the AHCA is a nonprofit federation of affiliated state health organizations, together representing more than 11,000 nonprofit and for-profit nursing facility, assisted living, developmentally disabled, and sub-acute care providers that care for approximately 1 million elderly and disabled individuals each day.

According to Federal Election Commission data, the AHCA Political Action Committee (PAC) contributed $1,298,000 to federal election candidate campaign committees between January 1, 2015 and December 31, 2016.

Examples of various AHCA contributions include $10,000 in 2014 to Senate Health, Education, Labor, and Pensions committee Chairman Senator Lamar Alexander (R-TN) and $8,000 in 2015 to ranking committee member Senator Patty Murray (D-WA). Also, committee member Senator Robert P. Casey Jr. (D-PA), who co-sponsored the request for a GAO audit of the Five-Star rating system for nursing homes, received a total of $11,000 in 2011, 2012, and 2014. Senator Ron Wyden (D-OR), a co-requester of the GAO audit with Casey, received a total of $7,500 from the AHCA PAC in 2013 and 2016.

In June 2015, the AHCA and the National Center for Assisted Living (AHCA/NCAL) gathered more than 400 long-term and post-acute care professionals at its annual congressional briefing event "to take the profession's legislative priorities to Capitol Hill, including progress and new goals within quality."

"Members of Congress tell us they want to hear directly from constituents, so our members have come to Washington to make sure our voice is heard," said AHCA/NCAL President and CEO Parkinson in a news

Chapter 13: Complaints Up; Enforcement Down

release. *"We will knock on the doors of Congress. We will make sure the message is clear. And we will continue our work to improve lives by delivering solutions for quality care."*

The news release continued:

"AHCA/NCAL members will share their professional experiences and discuss several topics of importance to long-term and post-acute care providers, including:

"--significant gains in the quality of care provided in skilled nursing centers and assisted living communities;

"--new AHCA/NCAL Quality Initiative goals;

"--thin operating margins for providers across the country;

"--counting observation stays in the hospital towards Medicare's required 3-day stay in order to cover skilled nursing care following a hospital stay.

"We must continue to have a visible presence in Washington and stand strong on the many issues that impact our profession."

The organization reported 400 health care professionals also participated in its 2016 event. The 2017 event was scheduled for June 5-6.

I invited AHCA to comment on an outline and selected notable issues from this book, posted on my website, in June 2017. Beth Martino, senior vice president for public affairs, AHCA, replied:

"Regarding your request to comment on specific issues in your book, as you already know from your research, skilled nursing and assisted living centers comply with

Chapter 13: Complaints Up; Enforcement Down

numerous regulations, along with state and federal laws, that protect our residents. Providing quality care to every resident is a top priority for our members. In addition, our members are committed to ensuring the safety and well-being of our residents. As an association, our focus is delivering resources to help centers provide quality care."

The AHCA website Fast Facts page on May 17, 2016 said there were 15,655 skilled nursing care centers with a total of 1.7 million beds in the U.S. It said 22 percent of individuals served were residing for short stays and 78 percent were residing for long stays, defined at 100 days or more. Forty-four percent of the residents were receiving post-acute (post-hospital) rehabilitation care.

The number of industry employees reported by AHCA was 1.7 million, of whom 1.2 million were health care practitioners and health care support workers; 387,000 were ancillary staff; and 162,000 were administrative staff.

AHCA said 57 percent of the cost of its services was paid by Medicaid, 14 percent by Medicare, and 29 percent by private insurance plans, other payers, and private individuals.

A March 2016 Industry Market Research Report by IBIS*World* estimated annual revenue of nursing care facilities in the US at $132 billion, for 24,115 businesses with 1.78 million employees.

Chapter 14:
Nursing Home Quality Improvement Task Force Report; "1-Hour Waits for Call Bell Responses"

After former Pennsylvania Attorney General Kathleen Kane filed a lawsuit against the Golden Living nursing home chain on July 1, 2015, alleging its nursing homes failed to provide the basic services for which customers, including the state, were paying, then-newly appointed Pennsylvania Secretary of Health Dr. Karen Murphy, PhD, announced on August 5, 2015, that she was forming a nursing home task force.

"I was deeply disturbed by these allegations regarding some Pennsylvania nursing homes and said we would take immediate steps to address the situation," said Murphy. "Today I am pleased to announce the Department of Health (DOH) has formed a task force to determine what

Chapter 14: Task Force Report; Resident Survey

additional measures can be taken to ensure enhanced quality in these facilities."

At one point, the task force's report was scheduled for release in June, 2016. I periodically inquired about the report, and was given target release dates that were further and further into the future. Finally, on September 26, 2016, a special assistant in the office of Secretary Murphy, with which I had been corresponding since February 2016, wrote and said: "We are looking to publicly release the report next week. I will make sure you get a copy! Thanks."

The DOH never sent me a copy. When I finally obtained one elsewhere early in October, I noted that its cover was dated September 22, 2016, 4 days before the special assistant promised to send me a copy "next week." I wondered whether state officials were reluctant to publicize the complete contents of the report, so they put out a summary of it in a news release.

The DOH issued an upbeat news release on October 4 stating: "Pennsylvania Department of Health Secretary Dr. Karen Murphy today released the recommendations of the Nursing Home Quality Improvement Task Force. The task force was created as part of the department's proactive efforts under the (Governor) Wolf Administration to make the most significant changes to nursing home oversight in nearly 2 decades."

The news release said the task force study would result in a "philosophical shift in regulations" that "will change how nursing homes function and improve the quality of life for all residents."

The news release said the task force "identified the following key areas in which to focus efforts:

Chapter 14: Task Force Report; Resident Survey

- "Improve collaboration between policy makers, lawmakers, providers, health care professionals, and most importantly, the residents of nursing homes and their advocates;
- "Change regulations and expand facility inspections to focus on the quality of life for residents who live in that facility;
- "Perform more comprehensive and consistent surveys to collect data that allows for consistent evaluation of quality of life in nursing homes; and
- "Redesign workforce composition and competencies."

I saw that the news release did not mention an 8-page section in the task force report that provided the results of a resident focus-group-style survey done at the request of the task force by the Pennsylvania Ombudsman Program.

In the survey, residents answered 12 questions about nursing home life in Pennsylvania. The first question was: "How satisfied are you with the quality of the physical care provided?" Sixty-two percent of the residents surveyed responded that they were "Very dissatisfied." Twenty-four percent said they were "Satisfied," and 14 percent said they were "Very satisfied." This information was not in the news release.

I observed that some of the conditions described in the survey were reminiscent of conditions my mother had experienced 5 years earlier. I was surprised that residents were complaining that it took an average of 45 minutes to 1 hour for nursing home staff to respond when a resident pushed his or her call button – a most basic component of nursing home care, and arguably the most important. I wondered if I was wrong to think this response time was disturbing.

Chapter 14: Task Force Report; Resident Survey

I felt that if the residents had taken the trouble to participate in the survey, at the request of the task force, their comments should have been summarized, or at least mentioned, in the press release. When I searched online for news stories about the task force report, none of the first 10 stories I found mentioned the resident survey. I did not look any further. The news stories I found were from media in parts of the country as widespread as Lancaster, PA, Montgomery, AL, and Oklahoma City, OK. I decided to include the comments of the nursing home residents in this book, so that the residents' voices might receive more attention. The entire survey report is printed at the end of this chapter.

An ombudsman who helped put the survey together told me: "Please do keep in mind that this was a small sample and a non-scientific survey. We did our best to quantitate anecdotal information provided to us by the residents. We felt it was a start to a more detailed dialogue on quality of care/quality of life in long-term care here in PA."

The task force report included a statement: "As the task force explored ways to better serve Pennsylvania's long-term care consumers, it was imperative that consumer [nursing home residents'] perspective be included in their comprehensive review."

The goal of the task force was to review regulations and identify areas that the department could improve.

In addition to members of the Governor's Office, and the secretaries of the Pennsylvania Departments of Aging, Human Services, and State, the task force members consisted of five PhDs, two MDs, a state senator, and a state representative.

Chapter 14: Task Force Report; Resident Survey

"Since coming into office, the Wolf Administration has made several significant changes to the Department of Health's nursing home care oversight to ensure we are doing our utmost to protect residents," said Secretary Murphy in her October 4, 2016 news conference announcing the task force report. "The task force helped us look at how we, as regulators, can improve our interaction with nursing homes, as well as the revisions that need to be made to the regulations themselves to improve the quality of life for all residents."

She said the task force confirmed a misalignment between outdated nursing home care regulations and the type of care that is needed in today's nursing homes. The task force concluded that in the past, state regulations were designed to evaluate the quality of the actual nursing home facility, but did not fully account for the quality of life of the residents themselves.

"Another important distinction to note is that a generation ago, a nursing home was a place to live out your final days," Secretary Murphy added. "Today, in addition to providing long-term care, nursing homes have become a place for short-term stays for the elderly following surgery or a prolonged hospital stay. We need to revise regulations to meet the needs of all nursing home residents."

In 2015, Murphy asked Auditor General Eugene DePasquale to take a critical look at how the state responds to nursing home complaints. His report highlighted three key areas where improvement was needed:

- Consistency when evaluating nursing homes' compliance with current staffing requirements;
- Procedures to respond to all complaints; and
- Effective methods to fine facilities that are out of compliance.

Chapter 14: Task Force Report; Resident Survey

These are discussed in Chapter 11.

The news release about the task force report listed improvements in oversight "since the beginning of the Wolf Administration." These were presented earlier in Chapter 9.

Responding to the task force report, the Pennsylvania Health Care Association (PHCA) said the report does not address human and financial resources needed for implementation.

W. Russell McDaid, president and CEO of the PHCA, an organization of nursing home providers, said in a statement:

"PHCA applauds the Pennsylvania Nursing Home Quality Improvement Task Force for their extensive work over the past 15 months to advance quality improvement in long-term care facilities across Pennsylvania, and we embrace the overarching goals set out for nursing home care in the seven specific recommendations outlined in the report.

"Pennsylvania's population is aging rapidly and the demand for long-term care services is growing, especially among residents and patients who have higher acuity levels, more complex medical needs, and chronic health conditions that require around-the-clock care.

"Pennsylvania's skilled nursing facilities fully support the three core components of the ideal care setting – quality of care, quality of living, and person-centered care. However, there are times when the voluminous state and federal regulations that govern nursing homes are in direct conflict with or limit a home's ability to fully embrace these core concepts.

Chapter 14: Task Force Report; Resident Survey

"One of the biggest challenges the Commonwealth will face in implementing these recommendations is the availability of resources—both human and financial.

"While the report acknowledges the current gap between Medicaid reimbursement and the full cost of compliance with the regulations governing nursing homes, it does not contain a single recommendation on how to close that gap, currently over $25 per Medicaid resident-day in Pennsylvania. Nor does it address a tort environment that is draining $95 million annually from the cash-strapped Medicaid program essentially to pay out-of-state attorneys who file frivolous lawsuits. These points must be part of the solution to protect seniors and help the state's fiscal situation."

The comment about the tort environment draining funds was an apparent reference to lawsuits by private individuals as well as three large ones filed by the Pennsylvania attorney general against nursing homes in collaboration with a Washington, DC law firm. These are discussed in Chapter 10.

The PHCA news release continued:

"Implementing the type of sweeping changes recommended in the task force report without dedicating additional state funding to pay for the increased costs that will be associated with the recommendations will further strain the finances of Pennsylvania's nursing homes, impacting nursing home residents and direct care workers by taking even more dollars away from the resident's bedside, where they are needed the most."

".... As we discuss changes to the regulations, Pennsylvania's dialogue must include a frank discussion of the availability of a competent, highly skilled workforce,

Chapter 14: Task Force Report; Resident Survey

and the financial resources necessary to pay and train them.

"Secretary Murphy noted that the Department has increased enforcement of regulatory sanctions and revised its calculations for how facilities are fined. It is important to note that more stringent penalties do not alone improve care. When any sanction or penalty is considered, the most important goal is to identify the practice in question, take steps to correct the practice, and ensure that any sanction does not jeopardize the facility's ability to improve resident care, comfort, and safety. Taking financial resources away from the bedside does not improve resident care.

"Despite chronic financial challenges, Pennsylvania's skilled nursing facilities have made strides in quality of care being provided with a focus on enhancing treatment services and improving the overall experience for residents, while improving in clinical outcomes, with reductions of urinary tract infections, pressure ulcers, use of antipsychotic medication, resident pain, and more."

Chapter 14: Task Force Report; Resident Survey

Nursing Home Quality Improvement Task Force Resident Survey Summary
Released October 4, 2016

(The following survey summary is reprinted verbatim, except for charts. Data from charts has been converted to text, with clarification where necessary. The entire task force report is on my website at https://www.wbeerman.com)

Background: The Pennsylvania Ombudsman Program was tasked by the statewide Nursing Home Quality Improvement Task Force to facilitate a survey of nursing home residents for purposes of gathering resident perspective and feedback regarding quality of life and quality of care measures in Pennsylvania.

Currently, there is a nationwide rating system (Five-Star Quality Rating System) in place for such a purpose. However, the existing rating system is based on clinical measures and provider self-reporting. As the Task Force explored ways to better serve Pennsylvania's long-term care consumers, it was imperative that consumer perspective be included in their comprehensive review.

The Pennsylvania Long-Term Care Ombudsman Program has a statewide network of consumers who have successfully completed a standardized, 10-hour curriculum intended to empower and educate them in topics including resident rights, state and federal licensing regulations, and self-advocacy skills and strategies. These residents are known as Pennsylvania's Empowered Expert Residents (PEERs.)

Since 2002, the PEER program has trained and graduated more than 3,000 PEERs. There is an existing network of approximately 1,190 PEERs at the time of this writing.

Chapter 14: Task Force Report; Resident Survey

The PEERs were eager to participate in the discovery process of this survey. Six resident meetings were convened in six homes across the state – all at a facility with a PEER presence.

Two meetings were held in each of our western, central, and eastern regions, and, for comparison, the two facilities selected in each region were on the opposite end of the spectrum of the Five-Star Quality Rating System.

Facilities ranged in size from a bed count of 51 to a capacity of 371 beds.

The sample included 29 residents, who varied in age and number of years living in the facility as outlined in the demographics section of this summary.

The intent of the survey was to compare and contrast the residents' experience with the Five-Star Quality Rating assigned to their respective facility.

Demographics:

Total Survey Responders: 29.

Total Number of Facilities: 6.

Resident Gender: Female, 59 percent; Male 41, percent.

Resident Age: 60 and older, 93 percent; 59 and younger, 7 percent.

Financial Structure: For-profit nursing home, 50 percent; nonprofit nursing home, 50 percent.

Comparative Length of Stay of Respondents: 13, or 50 percent, 0-2 years; 9, or 30 percent, 2-4 years; and 7, or 20 percent, 4-10 years.

Circumstances Possibly Impacting Accuracy of Data:

There were two interviewers/facilitators involved, and the style of the discussions may not have been identical. However, the questions used with each group were standardized and approved by the task force prior to the beginning of the group meetings.

The residents involved were also unfamiliar with their respective facilitator/interviewer, but each group included the local ombudsman, who did have an established relationship with the PEERs involved.

Finally, it is important to note that quality of life and quality of care are subjective matters. Each individual has preferences and priorities and individualized experiences that color his/her opinion regarding the overall quality of the facility where he/she resides.

The questions were open-ended and produced narrative and anecdotal responses. For the purposes of this summary, like answers are grouped and trends are identified as much as possible.

Question 1: How satisfied are you with the quality of the physical care provided?

Very satisfied, 14 percent; satisfied, 24 percent; very dissatisfied, 62 percent.

• The size and financial structure of the home appeared to be a factor in the response to this question. In general, satisfaction decreased with the increased size of the home (i.e., bed count).

• The time of day when assistance is requested also is a variable that impacts perception of quality. All residents reported that availability of help/response to requests for assistance vary based on shift and days of the week. For instance, residents who were generally satisfied did report

Chapter 14: Task Force Report; Resident Survey

that they can be very dissatisfied on overnights and weekends. Resident acuity also impacted this measure – the more help that is required (two staff members versus one, for instance), the harder it is to secure help and to feel safe and comfortable in the help provided. Residents attributed this to the number of staff assigned versus the number of staff needed to provide all residents with the care they need.

- Residents overwhelmingly agreed that the current resident-to-staff ratio is inadequate.

- Staff often get impatient with residents and appear rushed/pressured to move and perform tasks quickly in order to accomplish everything assigned to them.

- Residents expressed concerns regarding infection control – especially in the shower area and with personal care. They often observe staff "cutting corners" or "skipping steps" in the interest of time. One resident, who is rehabilitating after an amputation, reported refusing showers due to this type of concern. He reports that the common shower area with residents "wheeled in/wheeled out" without cleaning between residents concerns him.

- There is a prevalent opinion that call bell response times are too lengthy and residents reported waiting an average of 45 minutes to 1 hour for a call bell to be answered – especially on evenings, nights, and weekends. Several residents reported that they have attempted to help themselves/taken risks to avoid an incontinent episode when staff is unresponsive to their call bell.

- Four of the six homes reported that showers have been cancelled by staff due to staffing-related issues, yet the residents assert that this reasoning is not accurately reflected in their medical record. For instance, at care plan meetings, they may be asked why they are refusing showers – when they are not refusing at all.

- Some of the residents reported that they have used their personal phone to call the front desk or their family when they have been unsuccessful in obtaining help on their own.

- Residents reported that they have experienced staff coming into their room, turning off the call bell, indicating that they will be right back and then not returning/failing to provide the care. Residents also reported that they have had staff pretend not to hear them or see their light in an attempt to avoid helping them.

- A few of the residents have overheard staff arguing about who was going to have to take care of them. Residents report feeling embarrassed as a result; this impacts their dignity and ability to feel cared for in their home.

Question 2: Do you feel your social and emotional needs are being met?

Yes, 52 percent; no, 48 percent.

Problematic areas:

- Independent access to outdoor areas/community is limited.

- Wander-guards and hall passes are required of all residents to leave the building, even when cognitive impairment is not present. Residents feel "controlled."

- Email and phone access ranges from none to fair for most residents. Residents with availability of funds can afford a phone/tablet/Internet. For those who are on MA (medical assistance) and receive the monthly PNA (personal needs allowance), they use shared equipment that is often not functioning or is difficult to access/lacks privacy.

- Transportation to non-medical appointments/outside activities has been discontinued at four of the six homes involved in this survey, making it very difficult for residents to remain connected to the community beyond the facility and interfering with relationships in their communities.

- PNA impacts ability to connect with the community as well. When a facility offers a trip to the mall (or something similar), residents often have no money to participate. One resident reported that he is having his television disconnected because he can no longer afford the monthly cable fee.

- Residents expressed an interest in facility-based classes on using Internet, Skype, Facebook, and other social media as a means to connect with community.

Question 3: Do you feel you are in charge of your own care?

Yes, 79 percent; no, 21 percent.

Problematic areas/points of particular interest:

- Residents in two of the six homes indicated that they are engaged in the care plan process, resulting in an increased ability to direct their care.

- Residents want direct, regular, and timely access to their physicians. Residents report that physicians rarely visit or, when they do visit, the meeting is very brief and lacks substance. Several residents reported that their medications have been started/changed/discontinued by their doctor – based solely on communication with the nurse. Residents are not always even aware that this type of conversation is occurring. Residents also remarked that the licensed nurses having these conversations with the physicians are the staff members who know them the least.

- Residents report that the staff most familiar with them are the nurse aides.

- Residents are regularly directed by facilities to utilize facility-affiliated providers instead of community-based providers in an attempt to reduce resident travel and related costs.

• Communication between disciplines and various licensed staff was typically described as poor, and most residents agreed that the lack of communication concerns them. It often manifests itself in missed appointments, for example.

• Not all residents have been invited to their care plan meetings. While they all know about the care plan process and their right to attend (via the PEER curriculum), obtaining details about the date/time of the meeting (to facilitate their participation) is often a challenging process.

• Medical test results are not regularly shared with the residents; many reported that they must ask or pursue results.

Question 4: What is one thing you would like to have known prior to admission?

• "What they tell you upon admission is not always true."

• "There wasn't enough staff to take care of me."

• "Resident rights are not always respected."

• "What was the real quality of care here?"

• "Other residents could get into my things."

Question 5: Did you choose the home where you reside?

Yes, 19 percent; No, 81 percent.

• Only 19 percent of the residents participating in the group discussions selected the facility where they are residing. Family and/or hospital staff made the selection and informed the residents where they would be going.

• Most did not have the opportunity to see the facility prior to admission.

- Most did not realize until after they were admitted that they had a right to decline or select for themselves.

Question 6: If you were administrator for 1 week what would you change?

Of the residents, 100 percent indicated that they would make changes. Common themes:

- Change the actual administrator and administrative staff; hire someone more compassionate.

- Maintain wheelchairs and make sure wheelchairs are cleaned; provide seating options beyond the two choices most have now: wheelchair or bed.

- Remediate feelings of powerlessness and improve respect for resident rights.

- Improve communication.

- Change menus; improve resident access to snacks.

- Improve overall atmosphere; add music and decorations and comfortable furniture, etc.

- "Staff would ask residents what they want – not tell residents what they have to do."

- Eliminate corporate menus and respond to resident meal requests.

- Improve resident access to private use of a telephone.

- "Add a bar; serve alcohol."

- Automate the entrance doors so residents can get in and out of the building.

- Create a conference room for resident use.

- Reduce background noise – alarms, loud televisions, paging, etc.

Chapter 14: Task Force Report; Resident Survey

Question 7: Do you feel safe here?

Yes, 52 percent; No, 48 percent.

Residents elaborated as follows:

• "I don't speak up because of fear; I often feel powerless, so I just go along."

• One resident reported actual harm that is under investigation by the Department of Health.

• Belongings are not safe and facilities do not make an effort to protect belongings/replace belongings that go missing.

• Some facilities seem to be admitting "anyone"; residents are encountering shackled/guarded residents in common areas – residents with acute mental health episodes, etc. Residents do not believe there is sufficient facility staff to keep them safe; they are unable to get help quickly via call bell.

• Staff seem to be short-tempered when rushed or forced to work overtime to cover for call-offs.

• A few residents reported that they have been scolded by staff; one resident actually stated she felt as though she deserved to be scolded. She said of herself, "I am a lot of work."

Question 8: How would you rate your facility: 1-star – 5-stars?

Facility 1, a religious nonprofit of approximately 50 residents, received a 5 from CMS, and a 5 from the residents.

Facility 2, a for-profit facility with approximately 125 residents, received a 1 from CMS and a 3.5 from the residents.

Facility 3, a nonprofit with approximately 300 residents, received a 4 from CMS and a 3.4 from the residents.

Facility 4, a for-profit with approximately 125 residents, received a 1 from CMS and a 1 from the residents.

Facility 5, a nonprofit with approximately 125 residents, received a 5 from CMS and a 3.7 from the residents.

Facility 6, a for-profit with approximately 150 residents, received a 1 from CMS and a 2.2 from the residents.

Question 9: If you had the chance to do it over again, would you still live here?

Yes, 64 percent; No, 36 percent.

Due to the apparent contradiction of the residents' previous statements and this answer, it was explored in more detail. Most residents expressed a willingness to "settle" rather than be moved and try to adjust all over again. Most were not willing to consider experiencing resettlement again.

Question 10: Does this feel like your home?

Yes, 55 percent; No, 39 percent; no answer, 6 percent.

Suggestions/comments from the residents:

- Improve ability for residents to navigate their environment. One resident reported that all the hallways look alike. "It is big and confusing, so I rarely try to venture off my unit."
- Improve lack of control over who becomes their roommate and lack of options when someone is incompatible. Most opt to stay in a less-than-pleasant situation rather than move out of the room they consider "theirs."
- Facility is not "clean/comfortable like my own home would be."

- "In my own home, I'd have my own phone, TV, pets."
- "I have no choice in décor; the common areas look like a hospital; there are no seasonal decorations."
- "Resident council is ineffective and staff fail to follow up on concerns."

Question 11: If you could change the laws and regulations, what would you change?

- Staffing, 31 percent.
- Physician services, 19 percent.
- Increase PNA, 16 percent.
- Activities/transportation, 13 percent.
- Rehab services, 9 percent.
- Availability of supplies, 6 percent.
- Training for staff, 6 percent.
- Availability of equipment: One resident reported that she requires a mechanical lift for transfers, and she always has to wait for two staff and a shared lift – increasing wait times for help.

Question 12: What is the difference between a good day and a bad day?

Resident comments:

- "When I have someone to talk to"
- "Staff who actually care"
- "Bingo"
- "A day without problems"
- "When I'm outside for fresh air"

Chapter 14: Task Force Report; Resident Survey

Summary:

Each group session required 2 to 2½ hours to complete. Several of the local ombudsmen involved in the process remarked that the type of questions and allotted time frame allowed for the residents to be more self-disclosing (compared to the resident meetings conducted during a Department of Health survey.)

The residents were all cognitively capable but were very clear in their concern for residents who cannot advocate for themselves or whom they perceive as more vulnerable.

The residents explained that it is often intimidating – and there are possible consequences – for speaking up to facility staff in regards to concerns. There seems to be a willingness to tolerate less-than-satisfactory care rather than risk making matters worse.

It should be noted that these residents, PEER graduates, are the residents who are best-positioned for self-resolution, so their inability to feel fully satisfied with their care is of noted interest to the Long-Term Care Ombudsman Program.

The residents were extremely grateful for the opportunity to share this important information with the Task Force. They felt they could do so without fear of retaliation and without concern that their reporting would result in a staff person being fired or disciplined. In addition, it was an important opportunity for the long-term care ombudsman program to learn how we can better serve the consumers who seek guidance from us.

Chapter 15: Advocates -- The National Consumer Voice for Quality Long-Term Care, and Problems with Nursing Home Closures

One might jump to a conclusion that the closure of a nursing home facing government regulatory pressure is a sign that regulations are being enforced effectively. But what if the closure seems to be a display of bungling and callousness? And what if the shutdown could have been avoided by routine continuous enforcement of regulations?

The National Consumer Voice for Quality Long-Term Care (LTC) distributed a 2016 study by Dr. Cynthia Rudder, PhD, called, "Successful Transitions: Reducing the negative impact of nursing home closures." Besides discussing more well-managed closures, the study described a horrendous closure in New York State, covered later in this chapter.

The Consumer Voice is the leading national voice representing consumers in issues related to LTC. The

Chapter 15 : Advocates, and Problems With Closures

organization tries to ensure that consumers are empowered to advocate for themselves. Consumer Voice is a primary source of information and tools for consumers, families, caregivers, advocates, and ombudsmen that can be used to help ensure quality care for the individual.

The National Consumer Voice for Quality Long-Term Care was formed as NCCNHR (National Citizens' Coalition for Nursing Home Reform) in 1975 because of public concern about substandard care in nursing homes. The Consumer Voice is the outgrowth of work first achieved by advocates working for Ralph Nader and later for the National Gray Panthers.

On its website, http://theconsumervoice.org/, Consumer Voice has a section called "Get Help," which helps users find an Ombudsman, Citizen Advocacy Group (CAG), or other LTC resources in their state or territory. CAGs are concerned citizens who advocate for quality LTC, services, support, and quality of life for residents and consumers in their locality, state, or region. The website has a section describing the role of the long-term care ombudsman.

Consumer Voice also publishes a book, *Nursing Homes – Getting Good Care There*, by Sarah Greene Burger, Virginia Fraser, Sara Hunt, and Barbara Frank. It is a how-to book and a "consumer action manual," and I wish I had known about it when my mother went to her nursing home. The outcome would have been different. Anyone reading my book needs to read the Consumer Voice book too, especially someone who is selecting a nursing home or already has someone in a nursing home. The second edition of the book was written in 2002, but reading it along with this one, readers will see that issues, unfortunately, have not changed much and *Nursing Homes – Getting Good*

Chapter 15 : Advocates, and Problems With Closures

Care There, is still current.

Another example of Consumer Voice's work is a webinar (seminar on the internet) series that it sponsors, such as one on March 8, 2017, in which it called attention to dangers that congressional deliberations on the American Health Care Act posed to long-term care consumers. The webinar also focused attention on proposed congressional limits on plaintiffs' awards in healthcare lawsuits.

The organization sponsored a webinar on October 21, 2016 about revisions to nursing home regulations issued by the Centers for Medicare & Medicaid Services (CMS).

The October 21 webinar presenters included Karen Tritz, director, Division of Nursing Homes, Survey and Certification Group, CMS; Eric Carlson, directing attorney, Justice in Aging; Toby Edelman, senior policy attorney, Center for Medicare Advocacy; and Robyn Grant, director of public policy and advocacy, Consumer Voice.

During the webinar, Director Tritz outlined newly released CMS regulation revisions and the other participants commented on them. Consumer Voice generally endorsed the regulation revisions, calling them "vital for nursing home residents." However, two major subjects of discussion were the absence from CMS regulations of (1) a numerical minimum staffing requirement for nursing homes, and (2) a requirement that a registered nurse be present 24 hours a day in nursing homes. The Consumer Voice organization and others contend CMS should include these requirements in CMS regulations.

The new CMS rule on staffing mandates that there be "sufficient" staff with appropriate competencies and skill

Chapter 15 : Advocates, and Problems With Closures

sets. Sufficiency of staffing will be determined by assessments of residents and individual plans of care, taking into consideration the number, acuity, and diagnoses of the facility's resident population in accordance with an assessment of the facility.

Consumer Voice supports a minimum staffing standard of 4.1 hours per resident day of direct care by nursing staff and certified nursing assistants. Pennsylvania, for example, has a numerical requirement of 2.7 hours per resident day, but the Pennsylvania health department can require a higher number for a particular nursing home if it deems necessary.

More information on CMS's 2016 rule changes follows later in this chapter.

Regarding the nursing home closure mentioned at the beginning of this chapter, Consumer Voice held a webinar on Dr. Rudder's study, which was funded by the Retirement Research Foundation, and distributed by Consumer Voice. The study was about vulnerable nursing home residents, who have already reluctantly left their homes, have become "dependent on others for all aspects of their lives," and are then forced to relocate when a nursing home closes.

Voluntary and involuntary nursing home closures are becoming more frequent, according to the study. "Nursing home closings can have serious negative effects on residents," the study report said. "Many residents experience transfer trauma. The response to the stress caused by a transfer or relocation may include depression, manifesting as agitation; increase in withdrawn behavior; self-care deficits; falls; and weight loss."

These negative effects, according to the study, "may be due to the fact that the closure of nursing homes seems to be inadequately addressed in state and federal laws and regulations and/or poor oversight and monitoring by states and the federal government."

The study report commented, "Failure to protect dependent nursing home residents in these crisis situations undermines the entire framework of nursing home resident protection established in federal law."

Some study participants said they felt that if enforcement actions were taken earlier and more consistently, care might improve before a facility has to close. Examples of early and more consistent enforcement cited by participants were: accurate citation of deficiencies and accurate categorization of deficiencies by scope and severity; imposition of the full range of available remedies; and holding providers accountable by requiring development and implementation of meaningful plans of correction to address deficiencies.

In addition to case studies of better handling of closures, the report cited a case study of the March 2014 closure of a home called Blossom South, in Rochester, Monroe County, NY. The report said Blossom South was known as a chronic underperformer, and obtained 98 percent of its revenue from its 161 beds from Medicaid. The study report said that during a 3- to 5-year span, staff changes of 11 social workers, 13 administrators, and eight directors of nursing had occurred at Blossom South. The facility had a history of poor surveys and went through 18 Department of Health inspections between 2010 and 2013 that resulted in multiple citations, the report said.

Chapter 15 : Advocates, and Problems With Closures

Blossom South was under the threat of involuntary closure for more than 6 months, but 2 days before the provider's agreement with CMS ended on March 16, 2014, the state informed Blossom there would be no more delays of closure.

At the time of the actual closing, 68 residents remained. Many were targeted to go to a facility in Utica, 130 miles east of Rochester. The destination home, which transferees did not choose, was a one-star nursing home, listed as "much below average" in inspections, staffing, and quality measures, the report said. The destination home was owned by a man whose name was still on Blossom South's license, the report said.

One paragraph in the report said:

"On March 16th, when arriving at the facility for his regular weekly visit, the ombudsman volunteer witnessed about nine vans outside the facility. Twenty-seven residents were being packed into the vans without their belongings. Residents told the volunteer ombudsman they did not know where they were going except they had heard Utica, NY mentioned. In the days after the transition, the local ombudsman program received multiple calls from upset family members about their loved ones being moved to Utica. Families stated that residents did not have their personal belongings, including one gentleman who was reportedly sent to the new facility without his prosthetic leg."

The report included a collection of quotes from closure observers:

"...resident belongings being trashed-bagged up with no labels as to whom it belongs."

Chapter 15 : Advocates, and Problems With Closures

"Possessions, chart and meds not going with resident."

"Resident sent without proper discharge paperwork."

"Moving day chaos."

"Families not knowing where residents are moved."

"The closure was one of the worst experiences of my life."

The report said: "After going through many years of poor care at Blosson South and then a disastrous transition, many residents ended up far from their family and community in other poorly performing nursing homes. According to the report:

- 58 residents left Monroe County – 27 to a one-star facility 130 miles away from family and friends.
- 35 residents stayed within Monroe County: 20 were placed in nursing homes and 15 were discharged to the community.
- Of the 20 placed in Monroe County nursing homes, all were sent to facilities with poor care and the same or mutual owners. One receiving facility was going through bankruptcy."

The report contained 61 recommendations for improving the nursing home closure process, including some recommendations for CMS, some for state regulatory agencies, and some for long-term care ombudsmen.

One of the findings in the report was that some state survey directors who participated in closures felt closures were successful. The report said:

"Unlike the ombudsmen, advocates, family members, and residents, 4 of the 6 survey directors who responded to

Chapter 15 : Advocates, and Problems With Closures

their anonymous on-line survey did not find any of the closures problematic except for unreasonableness of residents and families. They did not seem to see success in the same way as the ombudsmen, advocates, residents, and family members did. They felt transitions were successful even if the residents and families were not happy about their new placement."

I solicited comments from a former managing partner of Blossom South, through his former or current attorneys, and from the New York Department of Health, through the governor's press office. No replies were forthcoming.

The Consumer Voice website has an online library, a news compendium, a listing of pertinent events and issues, and a support section containing information about program management, program promotion, training, systemic advocacy, and volunteer management.

The organization holds a major conference in Washington, DC each year.

In a statement released December 15, 2016, Consumer Voice said:

"This statement has epitomized the work of Consumer Voice this past year. Bringing the voice of the consumer to the policy table has been at the heart of our efforts as we:

- Work to educate and equip consumers, ombudsmen, and other advocates about newly released revisions to federal nursing home rules, the first widespread revisions in nearly 25 years;
- Support and engage our newly formed Consumer Advisory Council, made up exclusively of individuals receiving long-term care and services in nursing homes, assisted living facilities, and home care settings;

Chapter 15 : Advocates, and Problems With Closures

- Advocated for nursing home regulations that better protect consumers, including banning of pre-dispute arbitration provisions in nursing home admission agreements;
- Coordinated a meeting between 25 current and former residents of long-term care facilities with representatives from federal agencies such as the Centers for Medicare & Medicaid Services, the Administration for Community Living, the Department of Justice, the Consumer Financial Protection Bureau, and the Social Security Administration;
- Address consumer concerns about nursing home enforcement and implementation of the Medicaid home- and community-based services rules in regular calls with federal officials;
- Advocated with Congressional staff for strengthened Ombudsman provisions in the Older Americans Act reauthorization and increased funding for Ombudsman programs.

"Our dedicated staff works tirelessly on these and many other efforts to promote and protect the rights and interests of consumers...."

As President-elect Trump was calling for a reduction in government regulations, Consumer Voice, in partnership with the organization, Justice in Aging, issued a fact sheet listing reasons why September 2016 revisions to CMS regulations were "vital for nursing home residents." The fact sheet list of regulation revisions and comments on them follows.

- Greater focus on addressing a resident's individual needs and preferences. A nursing home must learn

more about who the resident is as a person, provide greater support for resident preferences, and give residents increased control and choice.
- Prompt development of a care plan. The original regulations allowed a resident to be without a care plan for as long as 21 days following admission. Now, a facility must develop and implement a care plan within 48 hours of a resident's admission.
- More comprehensive care. Treatment and services have been expanded to include pain management, dialysis, and behavioral health services.
- Improved training. Training requirements have been expanded to apply to all staff, contractual employees, and volunteers. Mandatory topics include communication, residents' rights, and prevention of abuse, neglect, and exploitation. Training for nursing assistants is expanded to include dementia management and resident abuse prevention.
- Improved protections against abuse, neglect, and exploitation. A nursing home must not employ a licensed individual with a disciplinary action, and must report suspicions of a crime to law enforcement and the state survey and certification agency.
- Better protection of resident property. Nursing homes are now required to take reasonable care of resident belongings and can no longer seek waivers of their responsibility for lost or stolen property.
- Increased visitation rights. A resident can accept visitors at any time of the day.
- Protection against evictions. Eviction for non-payment is not allowed when a third party payor (such as Medicaid) is evaluating a claim for payment. For evictions based on a nursing home's

Chapter 15 : Advocates, and Problems With Closures

supposed inability to meet a resident's needs, the nursing home must document its attempts to meet the resident's needs, and the ability of a receiving nursing home to meet those needs.
- Limiting nursing home's ability to "dump" a resident at the hospital. In an effort to evade eviction safeguards, some nursing homes "dump" residents by refusing to readmit them from hospitalizations. Now, a nursing home must follow eviction procedures and give a hospitalized resident an opportunity to appeal, when the nursing home claims that the resident cannot return.
- Prohibiting forced arbitration of claims of misconduct. Currently, many nursing home admission agreements compel a resident to bring any future claims about abuse, neglect or other quality of care issues through private arbitration. The revised regulations prohibit nursing homes from forcing residents to arbitrate disputes, but allow voluntary arbitration agreed to after a dispute arises. (This regulation revision was the subject of a legal challenge at the time this book was published.)

On April 11, 2017, a statement entitled: *Urgent Need for Effective Oversight to Counter Persistent Abuse and Neglect of Nursing Home Residents,* was issued by Richard Mollot, executive director of the Long Term Care Community Coalition (LTCCC); Lori Smetanka, executive director, and Robyn Grant, director of public policy and advocacy, for Consumer Voice; Toby Edelman, senior policy attorney for the Center for Medicare Advocacy; and Patricia McGinnis, executive director, Michael Connors, advocate, and Janet Wells, public policy consultant, for the California Advocates for Nursing Home Reform.

The five-page statement cited various evidence that

nursing home abuse, neglect, and substandard care persist at unacceptable levels but accountability for meeting minimum standards has decreased.

For example, LTCCC cited data in a February 2017 report by the non-profit Voices for Quality Care, that 42 percent of U.S. nursing homes, or 6,000 homes, have what LTCCC called chronic deficiencies in care. Chronic deficiencies were defined as three or more repeat citations for the same safety standard in a 3-year period. The Social Security Act requires that "any nursing home that does not achieve substantial compliance with the Federal requirements within six months be terminated from participation in Medicare and/or Medicaid," LTCCC pointed out.

The statement also said that according to https://data.medicare.gov, fines levied upon nursing homes decreased 9.83 percent from $57.2 million in 2015 to $51.6 million in 2016.

Epilogue:
The Need for Constant Vigilance; "Residents Still in Jeopardy"

"The price of liberty is eternal vigilance," said Thomas Jefferson.

Similarly, constant vigilance is necessary to protect nursing home residents from neglect and mistreatment, which have been recurring and persistent problems.

Some facts regarding nursing home oversight raise the question: **"Are residents still in jeopardy?"** For example, this book has performance charts showing clearly that some trends regarding nursing home oversight have gone in the wrong direction in recent years.

Ironically, numbers of consumer complaints about nursing homes have increased substantially while government oversight agencies have been issuing fewer citations for serious deficiencies and taking fewer enforcement actions.

To take a brief look back, in March 1998, then Pennsylvania Auditor General Robert P. Casey, Jr., (D) now a U.S. senator, released an audit report about the Pennsylvania Department of Health's (DOH's) oversight of

Epilogue: Residents Still in Jeopardy

nursing homes. It was entitled, "Residents in Jeopardy." Shortly thereafter, he released another audit report on the same subject, aptly entitled, "Residents Still in Jeopardy."

In a 1998 news release referring to the two audits, Casey said the Pennsylvania DOH had "failed miserably" in its oversight of nursing home care and that audit findings were "alarming."

Casey cited statistics showing that in 1996 the DOH issued only 45 sanctions against nursing homes, 58 fewer than it issued in 1994, a year in which there were 41 fewer nursing homes in Pennsylvania. I myself found that, amazingly, in 2012, DOH took only <u>two</u> enforcement actions. Apparently, the heightened vigilance that followed the 1998 Casey audits faded away almost completely by 2012.

Evoking a sense of déjà vu, Auditor General Eugene A. DePasquale said in a July 2016 audit report: "By some standards, nursing home care in Pennsylvania is declining."

In 2012, after the death of my mother, Mary Regina, in August 2011, I suggested to a former Pennsylvania auditor general that he audit state government's oversight of nursing homes. I wrote, "I would be happy to provide details supporting a conclusion that the oversight is not effective, is a waste of money, and fails to protect nursing home residents."

In responding, a deputy auditor general referred me back to the Casey audits from the late 1990s. She pointed out that corrective actions were taken as a result of those audits. Also, she said, a "task force" was established to improve the oversight of nursing homes. She added, "Your suggestion that still more improvements are needed is one

Epilogue: Residents Still in Jeopardy

that I will keep on hand." She said my audit suggestion would be considered for inclusion in the next year's audit plan.

However, in the next year, a different auditor general took over the office. No significant audit of nursing home oversight in Pennsylvania was done between 2000 and 2015, when more sensational negative news about nursing homes erupted in the media and a newly appointed secretary of health requested an audit of the DOH.

I noted that in 2011 Mary Regina had fallen victim to some of the same problems disclosed by the 1998 audits. Neglect of dehydration contributed substantially to her downfall, as it had for a victim cited in a 1998 Casey audit. Casey in 1998 deplored the dehydration case as one of numerous examples of "late and lax investigations of life-threatening nursing home complaints." Also, in 2011 Mary Regina and I had not been able to obtain enough information to properly choose a nursing home. That problem had been cited in a 1998 audit as well.

Further, as noted, the DOH issued only two enforcement actions for the entire year of 2012, the year of my official complaint about my mother's nursing home. The number was so unbelievably low that I had to ask the Office of the Secretary of Health to verify its accuracy. The office did verify it, in an email.

A chart in Chapter 9 of this book, provided by the secretary of health who took over the job in 2015, shows that enforcement actions in Pennsylvania generally trended down from 2002 until 2015.

On the national level, the Government Accountability Office (GAO) reported that the average number of consumer complaints filed per nursing home per year increased 21 percent from 2005 to 2014, while the number of serious deficiencies cited by inspectors/surveyors per nursing home surveyed per year <u>decreased</u> 41 percent over the same period.

The Centers for Medicare & Medicaid Services (CMS), which oversees nursing homes at the national level, also reported a decline in the average number of deficiencies cited per nursing home surveyed from 2006 to 2014.

A CMS official attributed the decline in citations largely to cuts in state oversight due to the "Great Recession," although other factors have been mentioned. Concerns also were being raised about the reliability of CMS's Five-Star Rating System for nursing homes, including issues raised in a December 2016 GAO audit report. The rating system did not consider the opinions of the people who were living in the nursing homes.

The national nursing home operators' association, which contributed $1,298,000 to federal election candidate campaign committees from January 1, 2015 through December 31, 2016, attributed the decline in deficiency citations to an improvement in care. The association also complained that nursing homes were overburdened with costly regulations, were plagued by allegedly unfounded lawsuits, and that Medicaid's payments were insufficient to cover the cost of care.

Meanwhile, the Pennsylvania attorney general alleged in a lawsuit filed in 2015 that some nursing homes in Pennsylvania, although "enormously profitable," were not adequately staffed to deliver the services they were getting paid for, and that nursing homes in many cases knew in advance when the state inspectors were coming for "unannounced" inspections.

Two consecutive attorneys general in New Mexico alleged in a suit similar to the Pennsylvania one that staffing in certain nursing homes was not adequate to provide the services for which the homes were billing. Pennsylvania and New Mexico attorney general suits were still ongoing in 2017. Suits filed by presumably unbiased government attorneys describe shocking conditions in nursing homes that allegedly resulted from inadequate staffing.

The current Pennsylvania auditor general, another presumably unbiased government official, said in an audit report in July 2016 that the DOH was not properly monitoring the staffing of nursing homes, at the same time evidence of poor resident care was being disclosed. The 2016 audit report also repeated the finding from 1998 that consumers were not getting enough information with which to choose a nursing home.

Two Pennsylvania newspaper reporters, Daniel Simmons-Ritchie and David Wenner, in a 2016 series of articles entitled "Failing the Frail," by PennLive.com/the *Patriot-News,* found that among 259 deaths due to serious incidents in Pennsylvania nursing homes from 2013 to 2015, nursing homes were cited by the DOH for a care-related death in only 46 cases. The state decided penalties were unnecessary in more than half of the 46 cases. The journalists said it was common for the DOH to understate the severity of deficiencies in fatal cases.

Epilogue: Residents Still in Jeopardy

Just as in 1998, a task force was established in 2015 in an effort to improve the quality of nursing home care and oversight in Pennsylvania. As part of its work, the task force commissioned a limited survey of nursing home residents to obtain their input for the task force report, which was published in October 2016. Among the findings of the focus-group-style survey, which included 29 residents from six representative nursing homes, was that 62 percent of the survey participants were "very dissatisfied" with the quality of physical care provided; they believed the staff-to-resident ratio was inadequate; and they waited an average of 45 minutes to 1 hour for responses to call bells.

Although I know that many people are working hard to improve nursing home care, I wonder whether some aspects of care have improved much since my mother was in a nursing home in 2011. I remember that response time to call bells was disgraceful in my mother's nursing home, but I do not remember it being as bad as an hour, as was indicated in the 2016 task force survey report.

I observed that quite a few nursing home residents must have endured almost incessant ringing of nurse call bells between 2011, when my mother complained of it, until 2016, when long waits for responses were cited in the Pennsylvania task force report. Mary Regina's nursing home was rated below average in 2011, and it was rated below average in 2016.

I remember that during my mother's stay in the nursing home, few residents seemed to get visitors. There also were few, if any, people to speak up for some residents.

Epilogue: Residents Still in Jeopardy

When the residents were asked as part of the 2016 task force survey, "What is the difference between a good day and a bad day," one responded: "When I have someone to talk to."

Notably, the survey of "what the residents think" was not mentioned in the Pennsylvania DOH's news release announcing the task force report, and the survey of what residents think got virtually no mention in the news media.

I found as I was working on this book that even as a former journalist whose book was likely to be circulated widely, I had difficulty getting government officials to respond to my inquiries. In some cases, I was told to submit Freedom of Information Act (FOIA) requests. It seemed that instead of facilitating citizens' access to public information, the FOIA created a virtual holding bin where citizens' requests for government information could be sent with impunity for indefinite periods instead of being answered.

I received a reply on May 2, 2017 to an FOIA request I had sent 8 months earlier on August 29, 2016 to the CMS FOIA officer. The response's 36-pages of information, some of which was not about nursing homes, did not seem to contain explicit answers to the four specific questions I asked in my FOIA request. (In fairness, I must say that three CMS officials were helpful to me in other matters over the course of my research. See Appendix E.)

In one case, questions I submitted to a senator in five different ways -- by email, paper mail, a web site, a fax, and telephone voicemail -- seemed to have been sent into a black hole on Capitol Hill. There was no reply at all.

Epilogue: Residents Still in Jeopardy

Meanwhile, it seemed to me that elected officials and agencies -- CMS, for example -- were well staffed and prolific at creating and issuing seemingly self-promotional, politicized, news releases that tout their purported successes. Many news releases praised the Affordable Care Act, even though popular opinion and the November 8, 2016 presidential election results seemed to indicate that the success of the Act was a debatable issue.

One CMS release on December 2, 2016 said per capita growth of health care spending "continues to be below the rates of most years prior to the passage of the Affordable Care Act." It quoted the acting CMS administrator as saying: "Our significant progress in reducing the nation's uninsured rate, while providing strong protections for Americans if they get sick, would not be possible without the Affordable Care Act." It added, "As millions more Americans have obtained health insurance, per-person cost growth remains at historically modest levels." I noted that the releases used vague words such as "most," "significant," "strong," and "historically modest."

A CMS news release headline on August 9, 2016 said: "Affordable Care Act payment model continues to improve care, lower costs." Two weeks later on August 25, 2016 a CMS news release carried the headline: "Physicians and health care providers continue to improve quality of care, lower costs."

Expressing an opposite view, President Donald Trump's eventual appointee as secretary of health and human services, physician Congressman Tom Price, said on October 25, 2016:

Epilogue: Residents Still in Jeopardy

"While President Obama and Democrats have the audacity to tout Obamacare's 'success,' the cold hard facts and figures prove the opposite is true. Every single day Obamacare is making the quality of health care in this country worse and next year alone, benchmark Obamacare premiums are set to increase 25 percent on average for states that use the federal healthcare market place."

Whatever one's political persuasion, the involvement of politics in health care, including nursing home care, should be quite evident.

One Democrat state auditor general actually was quoted in the Pennsylvania press as saying he thought a former Republican governor's administration banned acceptance of anonymous complaints about nursing homes "to silence critics." Enforcement actions were way down in the state under that governor's administration, as they were nationally under the most recent Democrat president.

Kathleen Kane, the elected Pennsylvania attorney general who at least appeared to be crusading for better nursing home care, was sentenced to 10-23 months in prison in October 2016. She had been convicted of perjury and of disclosing grand jury information to discredit a political enemy. Although an unusual case, it does not inspire confidence in government as an overseer of nursing home care.

Kane, a Democrat, was embroiled in political wars and claimed she was fighting a "good old boys" club. She was accused of stifling a corruption investigation of Democrat politicians that had been initiated by her Republican predecessor. A scandal Kane exposed about a pornography email network in state government touched officials in the

Epilogue: Residents Still in Jeopardy

Republican governor's office and reportedly led two state Supreme Court justices to resign. News coverage of the scandal included reports of infighting between individual Supreme Court justices themselves. As this book was being published, the Pennsylvania Supreme Court, which had lost two members to Kane's pornography expose', was adjudicating an appeal regarding a big nursing home lawsuit that Kane had filed before her demise.

Evidence of the interlacing of politics in nursing home oversight that is more obvious is the extent of political campaign contributions passing between health providers and elected officials, which is discussed in other parts of this book. An "obvious" example of the access the nursing home industry has to politicians is a June 12, 2017 news release photo of American Health Care Association President and CEO Mark Parkinson, a former governor of Kansas, and other AHCA officials, meeting with new U.S. Health and Human Services Secretary Price at HHS. The news release is posted on my website: https://www.wbeerman.com.

Government officials, such as governors, appoint those who run the agencies overseeing nursing homes. Some such appointees may not want to see the governor or some other official who appointed them be embarrassed by bad publicity about nursing homes. Most likely there is pressure to suppress nursing home scandals or spin the news. I wonder whether Kane's disclosure of embarrassing facts about state government's lax oversight of nursing homes helped foster political animosity toward her.

Kane's lawsuit disclosed suspicious circumstances surrounding allegations that a considerable number of

Epilogue: Residents Still in Jeopardy

nursing home managers knew when the government inspectors were coming for "unannounced" inspections.

On a tangential issue, HHS Secretary Price, a doctor who received almost a half-million dollars in campaign contributions from the health sector in 2015-2016, favors limiting potential jury awards to patients in health care cases as a way to keep costs down. The term, tort reform, being advocated as a part of health care reform, refers to proposed changes by legislators that aim to reduce the ability of victims to bring litigation or to reduce the damage awards they can receive.

In my experience, it was, and is, already difficult to undertake lawsuits on behalf of elderly victims of alleged health malpractice. Some lawyers, although not all (See Appendix D), see cases regarding elderly people as having low potential for substantial awards because older people, especially retired persons, do not lose many years of lifetime earnings potential, or even many years of life expectancy, when injured. Also, in many cases, Medicare and Medicaid must be repaid for their patient-care expenditures out of lawsuit settlement funds, which substantially decreases any award proceeds that may be left for the victim. This scenario is unfavorable for nursing home residents or their families who seek legal recourse.

Nevertheless, as detailed in the book, I found in my research that some lawyers -- state attorneys general, for example, and private-practice nursing home specialists – sometimes seem to have more success in holding nursing homes accountable than do government oversight agencies set up for that purpose. The attorneys are able to put to good use in court the records that government oversight

Epilogue: Residents Still in Jeopardy

agencies create through their inspections and administrative work.

On November 2, 2016, I heard a story that touched my heart. New Mexico Congressman Steve Pearce related in a speech that while he was flying a C-130 during the Vietnam War, he listened in on the radio as an American fighter jet with two crew members was shot down. The downed crew asked over the radio that they be picked up by a nearby rescue helicopter. One of the two was picked up -- he was in the water. The other crew member was on land.

"The Rules of Engagement required the rescue helicopter to get clearance to pick up the one who came down on land," recalled Pearce. "That clearance had to come from command headquarters in Hawaii. But darkness had set in before the clearance was received back from Hawaii. Throughout the night over the open mic, rescuers heard automatic weapons. The next morning, contact with the lone crew member was attempted, but fate had already decided his way."

This reminded me that just as the airman was a victim of a policy decision made remotely, people in all walks of life who are in need of rescue of some sort become victims of slow action, non-action, or bad decisions by government officials and employees. Many residents of nursing homes, like the one who said a good day is "when I have someone to talk to," suffer alone. As things stand now, one must wonder whether they will be rescued.

I noticed that much of the CMS management data about the performance of nursing homes and oversight

Epilogue: Residents Still in Jeopardy

agencies is a year old, or even much older, which may indicate slow processing.

Although in 2010 the Affordable Care Act added an enforcement requirement for CMS to establish an automated system for collecting payroll data on nurse staffing hours in nursing homes, that requirement still had not been fully implemented in mid-2016.

After members of Congress requested an audit of the Five-Star nursing home rating system in August 2015, the audit report did not come out until November 2016, which is not exceptionally slow for an audit report. The corrective actions recommended by the auditors routinely will come some time after the audit, if at all. Nevertheless, auditors, especially GAO, along with attorneys and advocacy organizations, seem to be among the best friends of nursing home residents.

Yet, 1 hour or 1 day, or 1 year or 5 years, can be a long time for someone suffering in a substandard nursing home and waiting to be rescued.

As this book was being prepared for publication, Congress was debating repeal and replacement of Obamacare, changes to Medicaid, and limits on healthcare litigation. The outcomes of these deliberations will have serious consequences for nursing home consumers.

Meanwhile, nursing home operators were contending that Medicaid payments were already $23-$25 per resident per day, or $7 billion per year nationally, short of what they needed to comply with standards of care.

Expecting that poor conditions in some nursing homes would not be corrected soon, I decided that I would plan to write a sequel to this book. For the sequel, I will solicit information from residents, nursing home staff, state enforcement staff, federal officials, and others about conditions in nursing homes. I especially would like to know whether consumers are happy with the way state agencies investigated their complaints.

So, interested persons are invited to provide information about the performance of oversight agencies, conditions in nursing homes, and efforts to improve conditions, for the sequel, at my web site, *https://www.wbeerman.com*.

Since information provided to me will be used only for the preparation of the sequel, I hope people will also report complaints to government agencies and seek help from advocacy organizations for nursing home residents such as those mentioned in Chapter 15, which may be able to provide timely help.

God willing, if I live long enough, I will publish a progress-report sequel sometime in the future. Maybe it will be called, "*Mary Regina's nursing home – Residents **Still** in Jeopardy*." But I hope I will be able to call it something different.

Appendix A: Master's Report

IN THE COURT OF COMMON PLEAS,
ALLEGHENY COUNTY, PENNA.

MASTER'S REPORT

DANIEL T. ZAMOS, ESQ

Mary R. Beerman, Plaintiff

Vs

William Beerman, Defendant,

In Divorce

DANIEL T. ZAMOS, ESQ., the Master appointed by the Court to take testimony of witnesses in the forgoing case and return the same together with report thereon, respectfully represents:

Appendix A: Master's Report

That pursuant to his appointment on January 23, 1969, the Master sat March 14, 1969, at 10:00 A.M., E.D.S.T, in the Court of Common Pleas of Allegheny County as the time and place of trial. Notice was given to ▮▮▮▮▮▮▮▮▮▮▮▮▮▮▮▮, ESQ., counsel for the plaintiff, and DENNIS C. HARRINGTON, ESQ., counsel for the defendant. Trial commenced at the time appointed and was concluded at 4:30 P.M. the same day.

I

SERVICE OF PROCESS

The complaint in this matter was filed on July 30, 1968, and a copy of the complaint together with Notice of Suit was served on the defendant personally on August 15, 1968.

II

GROUNDS FOR DIVORCE

1. Indignities

III

FINDINGS OF FACT

1. MARRIAGE: The parties were married May 21, 1947, in Allentown, Pennsylvania [Allentown is a neighborhood of Pittsburgh].

2. RESIDENCE AND JURISDICTION:

At the beginning of their marriage, the parties lived on Agnew Road, Baldwin Township. In September, 1950, the parties moved to a home they were buying at 1441 Washington Boulevard, Port Vue, Allegheny County, Pennsylvania, where they remained until their separation which precipitated their divorce action on June 23, 1968.

The plaintiff now lives at 1434 Tolma Avenue, Pittsburgh, Pennsylvania, with her parents. The defendant's current address was not determined by the testimony.

Appendix A: Master's Report

3. AGE AND OCCUPATION

The plaintiff is 44 years of age. She was not employed during the course of the marriage. The defendant's age was not brought out during the testimony though he apparently was approximately the same age as the plaintiff. Though he worked various jobs from time to time, the defendant was primarily employed as a steelworker during the marriage.

4. CHILDREN

Two children were born of the marriage: William John, 20, and Regina, 11.

5. FINDINGS ON MERIT AND DISCUSSION

1. The parties were married on May 21, 1947.
2. At the time of the marriage the defendant was employed at one of the local steel mills. The plaintiff was not employed.
3. The parties first lived together in an apartment rented from one ▬▬▬▬▬▬, a long-time friend of the defendant's. They lived there until they purchased a home which they now own in 1950, and in which the defendant is now residing; the plaintiff having left their common residence around July 27, 1968, after their estrangement became complete.

PLAINTIFF'S TESTIMONY

The chief complaint of the plaintiff is centered about:
a) The defendant's alleged infidelity and/or "improper" behavior with other women.
b) The defendant's failure to properly support the plaintiff and children.
c) Differences concerning the raising of their children.

A. ALLEGED INFIDELITIES OF THE DEFENDANT

1. The complaints concerning "other women" in the defendant's life centered about four specifically named women:

Appendix A: Master's Report

Mrs. ███████████, Mrs. ███████████, Mrs. ███████████, and a woman named ███.

2. The plaintiff testified that the parties quarreled about every two months concerning other women (N. T. p.7). That during one of their arguments over "girlfriends," she threw a cup of coffee at him and he struck her (N.T. p. 13). She said that the defendant would cause incidents that provoked the quarrels (N.T. p. 36).

3. The plaintiff testified that the defendant admitted sitting in a parked car with "███," a fellow employee from Capital TV where the defendant worked on a second job, and that he was told to move by the police (N.T. pp. 19, 20).

4. She testified that the defendant often visited Mrs. ███████████, the wife of their former landlord in the absence of her (███████)'s) husband (N.T. p. 20, 21, 22).

5. The plaintiff related that she was embarrassed and "went into a fit" by the defendant's dancing with one Mrs. ███████████, a mutual acquaintance, though the dancing was done in her (the plaintiff's) presence and that of Mrs. ███████'s husband (N.T. pp 23, 24, 25). She said that this happened on four or five occasions. The plaintiff, however, admitted to being jealous (N.T. p. 24).

6. Finally, the plaintiff contended that the defendant frequently was in the company of one Mrs. ███████████ on Sunday mornings after taking his boy to church (N. T. p. 27). She testified that her husband admitted "he was seeing this woman" (N. T. p. 28).

B. **FAILURE TO PROPERLY SUPPORT PLAINTIFF AND CHILDREN**

1. The plaintiff stated that on their return from their honeymoon the defendant informed her that his plant had shut down for a two-week period and that they had to move in with her parents for three weeks (N.T. p. 5). That her parents had to support them (N.T. p.5).

2. That from payday to payday they would run short of money and have to borrow from her parents, that this was

Appendix A: Master's Report

embarrassing to her, and that it continued for seventeen years (N.T. p. 6)

    3. She stated that the defendant lacked seniority where he worked and was often laid off because of this and frequent strikes (N.T. p. 11).

    4. But the plaintiff also complained that the defendant sometimes worked two jobs and that at one time worked eighteen hours a day, seven nights a week (N.T. p. 46)

C. DIFFERENCES IN CHILD RAISING.

    1. The only testimony given by the plaintiff in this regard was vague and general. She stated that the defendant did not believe in reprimanding a child excessively and that they quarreled frequently about this. (N.T. p. 11)

CROSS EXAMINATION OF THE PLAINTIFF ON:

A. ALLEGED INFIDELITIES:

    1. The plaintiff conceded that the worst thing she ever saw her husband do with ▓▓▓ was to dance with her in her presence and that of Mrs. ▓▓▓'s husband (N.T. pp. 76, 77). That she constantly reminded him of this (N. T. p. 75). But that he had no improper relationship with any woman for the last fifteen years of their marriage (N. T. p. 75). She admitted that all of the defendant's alleged improprieties with ▓▓▓ occurred in her presence (N. T. p. 103)

    2. The plaintiff admitted that all the defendant ever told her about his behavior with ▓▓▓ was that he visited her and nothing more (N. T. p. 102).

    3. Much of what the plaintiff accused the defendant was based on hearsay from a Mrs. ▓▓▓ and from neighbors (N. T. pp. 94, 98). She made repeated accusations, nevertheless (N. T. pp. 92, 93, 94).

Appendix A: Master's Report

B. FAILURE TO SUPPORT

1. The plaintiff agreed that the defendant never quit a job to "loaf" (N. T. p. 58). That he worked overtime, took extra jobs, one at a gasoline station where he worked 800 hours in one year and always brought his money home (N.T. p. 59). She admitted that she handled all the money (N. T. p. 60). That he later provided the family with two cars, one for her use (N. T. p. 61). That he did all the shopping for the last twelve years of their marriage (N. T. p. 85). That he had no outside social life and spent most of his time working (N.T. p. 88). That only once while they were living together did they have to go on public assistance because the defendant was laid off from work. That this was embarrassing to her and that she never let him forget it (N. T. pp. 70, 71, 72).

C. DIFFERENCES REGARDING CHILD RAISING

1. The plaintiff admitted that the defendant ... showered a father's attention to his children N. T. pp. 70, 71, 72).

OTHER WITNESSES FOR PLAINTIFF

1. The plaintiff called a Mrs. ███████████ as her witness, but Mrs. ███'s testimony produced little, if anything, of probative value to the case.
2. She then called her mother, Mrs. John A. Fisher, who stated that the couple had borrowed money from her occasionally and that she bought clothes for her grandchildren (N.T. pp. 110, 111). She stated that she became aware of the parties' quarrels only during the last eight months of the marriage (N. T. p. 111).
3. Mr. John Fisher, the plaintiff's father, testified that the plaintiff complained of having to borrow money from him so often (N. T. p. 115). But that he never observed any misconduct on the part of her husband (N.T. p 117).

Appendix A: Master's Report

DEFENDANT'S CASE

1. The first witness called by the defendant was Mrs. ▮▮▮▮▮. She stated that she lived about ▮▮▮ from the Beermans (N.T. p. 122). That she was never in (Mr.) Beerman's company alone. That the only time she was in the Beerman home was to register them to vote and that she had seen Mr. Beerman only three or four times in eighteen years and had no idea what gave rise to Mrs. Beerman's accusations.

2. Her husband also testified that he could not account for Mrs. Beerman's accusations concerning his wife. That his wife did take their children to Mass on Sundays, come back home and return later to pick them up and that she would have no opportunity to go riding with him or visit Mr. Beerman (N. T. pp. 128, 129).

DEFENDANT'S TESTIMONY

1. The defendant testified that ▮▮▮▮▮▮▮▮ was a lifelong friend of his; that he and his wife lived in the ▮▮▮ home for a short period of time; that there was never any estrangement between them, and that they continued to be friends after he and his wife moved from their home (N. T. pp. 134, 135). He said that the plaintiff referred to his relationship with Mrs. ▮▮▮ during the entire period of their marriage (N. T. pp. 137, 138). That she made accusations concerning infidelities in front of the children (N. T. p. 141). He denied that there was anything between him and Mrs. ▮▮▮ or any other woman (N. T. pp. 135, 136, 137).

2. The defendant testified that the plaintiff finally quit talking to him, refused to make meals for the family, and would throw dishes into the garbage can. She told the defendant that she hated his guts and that all she wanted was "to get the hell out of this place," meaning their home (N. T. p. 149).

3. The defendant related the circumstances leading to the plaintiff's leaving their common domicile on July 27, 1968 (N. T. pp. 151, 152).

Appendix A: Master's Report

CONCLUSION

The plaintiff obviously was a high-strung, highly nervous individual who suffered some sort of physical affliction which was not fully determined. She was highly sensitive to the defendant's connection to any woman and showed extreme jealousy. The incidents related by her concerning other women were trivial, at best, and would hardly have affected the sensibilities of the average wife. She was highly embarrassed over minor financial matters without just cause. Rather than overlook these minor annoyances, she constantly referred to them during the entire marriage even though the causes had been removed more than fifteen years prior to the couple's separation. She failed to completely substantiate that the defendant's behavior with other women was out of the ordinary.

Though the plaintiff complained that the defendant did not properly provide for her and her family, she failed to prove this. The defendant was gainfully employed throughout most of the marriage, more often than not, working two jobs. He gave her his pay and she handled the money. They were able to buy a home of their own and own two cars during most of their married life.

It is the conclusion of the Master, therefore, that the plaintiff failed in her proof that the defendant subjected her to such indignities as would entitle her to a divorce.

CONCLUSION OF LAW

1. The plaintiff and defendant contracted a legal marriage which still exists.
2. The Court has perisdiction over both parties and subject matter.
3. There has been no fraud or collusion between the parties.
4. The plaintiff is not entitled to a divorce on the grounds of indignities.

Appendix A: Master's Report

Notices of the intention to file the report of the Master, a copy of which is attached hereto, have been forwarded to counsel of record of both parties.

RECOMMENDATION

In accordance with the Finding of Fact and Conclusions of Law, the Master respectfully recommends that a Divorce from Bed and Board be denied.

DANIEL T. ZAMOS
Master

Appendix B:
Amended Bill of Particulars

IN THE COURT OF COMMON PLEAS OF ALLEGENY COUNTY, PENNSYLVANIA

FAMILY DIVISION

MARY R. BEERMAN, Plaintiff

WILLIAM BEERMAN, Defendant

AMENDED BILL OF PARTICULARS

AND NOW comes the plaintiff, Mary R. Beerman, and herewith Amends the Bill of Particulars in this matter and substitutes the following in place thereof:

1. Immediately after the marriage of the Plaintiff and Defendant on May 21, 1947, the Plaintiff and Defendant were forced to live with the Plaintiff's parents for two or three weeks and Plaintiff was continually forced to accept charity from her parents and family, for the next 17 years.

Appendix B: Amended Bill of Particulars

2. The Plaintiff and the Defendant engaged in quarrels and arguments continuously during the course of their marriage concerning such subjects as: his running around with other women, the raising of their son, his refusal to seek work when he was unemployed.

3. The Defendant on numerous occasions threatened the Plaintiff with physical and/or bodily harm to her person, making menacing gestures and intimidating remarks, causing the Plaintiff to be in fear and a constant state of tension and anxiety concerning the possibilities of these threats being consummated into acts by the Defendant.

4. In 1950, the parties were forced to move from their place of residence on Agnew Road, Baldwin Township, Pennsylvania, by their landlord, ███████, because the landlord accused the Defendant of making illicit advances toward his wife, ███████, all of which the defendant boasted about in public.

5. In 1953 and the year following, the Defendant was employed as a television salesman with Capital TV and remained out for unreasonable lengths of time and at hours of the early morning on the pretext of working. During this employment the Defendant admitted to the Plaintiff that he had been keeping company with a woman named ███ and cited one example of being with her when the police forced them to move from an alley in which they were parked.

6. In 1956 six years after the Plaintiff and Defendant were forced to move from their place of residence in Baldwin, Plaintiff received a telephone call from her former landlord's wife, ███████, and ███████ informed the plaintiff that Defendant had just left her company, and that she could begin to prepare his

Appendix B: Amended Bill of Particulars

dinner. The defendant admitted visiting her periodically, in her husband's absence.

7. During the years 1954 and 1955 the Defendant did keep company with a woman named ▆▆▆▆▆▆▆, a neighbor of the parties, who would come to the residence of the parties on numerous occasions, clothed in her pajamas and ask to dance with the Defendant, and the Defendant condoned and encouraged such conduct in the presence of the Plaintiff.

8. In 1957, when the Plaintiff was pregnant with the daughter of the parties, the Defendant began to keep company with a woman named ▆▆▆▆▆▆▆, meeting with her at various times when he was, to the Plaintiff's knowledge, supposed to be in church with their son.

9. In September and October of 1963, the Plaintiff was confined to McKeesport Hospital for a female operation and the third day following the operation Defendant visited the Plaintiff and wanted sexual intercourse.

10. During Plaintiff's confinement in McKeesport Hospital during April, 1966, Defendant purposely and maliciously frustrated and upset the Plaintiff by informing the Plaintiff during visiting hours that:

> a. Plaintiff's daughter had appendicitis but the Defendant had not taken her to the hospital, or called a doctor;
>
> b. Defendant had sold Plaintiff's and Defendant's home;
>
> c. The Defendant had quit his job and as a result they had no money;

Appendix B: Amended Bill of Particulars

d. All of the above statements were untrue.

11. During the Plaintiff's confinement in McKeesport Hospital in April 1966, the Defendant's visits had an upsetting effect upon the Plaintiff because of the instances described in No. 10, and as a result the nurse suggested that the Plaintiff should inform her husband not to visit her any more.

12. For a period of approximately three years prior to April 1966, the Defendant had knowledge of the Plaintiff's weakened physical condition and maliciously complained that she was lazy.

13. In April of 1966, the Defendant was informed by the Plaintiff's doctor, James Harris, M.D., that the Plaintiff was suffering from Addison's disease and that she was not to be upset or frustrated unnecessarily and Defendant failed and refused to accept this advice and to the contrary, caused emotional disturbances to the Plaintiff.

14. For a great number of years the Defendant has threatened to throw the Plaintiff out of their home or leave himself and not allow her to have the children.

15. During each of the five occasions on which the Plaintiff was hospitalized, for various reasons including child birth, the Defendant failed to render to the Plaintiff the proper attention, sympathy and understanding of her physical problems.

16. During the entire course of their married life, the Defendant demanded [this nonmaterial allegation was withheld from the book to avoid offending some readers].

17. The Defendant never exhibited to the Plaintiff any compassion or consideration concerning the physical

Appendix B: Amended Bill of Particulars

condition from which she suffered, and refused and failed to render to her any comfort or support.

18. The Defendant, throughout the entire course of the marriage to the parties, caused the Plaintiff to be embarrassed and humiliated in front of other people.

19. The Defendant, throughout the entire course of the marriage of the parties, lied to the Plaintiff and deceived her in a great many ways.

20. From June 23, 1968 until January 21, 1969, the Defendant failed and refused to provide the Plaintiff with the financial means and resources to maintain herself and their daughter, in spite of the fact that the Defendant was fully employed and working two jobs for a period of 18 hours per day.

21. That the Defendant, by his failure and refusal to support and maintain the Plaintiff and his child since the parties have been separated in July, 1968, has caused the Plaintiff to become a public charge for her support and maintenance through the Department of Public Welfare of the Commonwealth of Pennsylvania, and caused the Plaintiff to accept gifts of charity in the form of clothing for their child, in order for her to return to school, in the fall of 1968, all of which has been the source of great embarrassment and humiliation to the Plaintiff.

22. On or about July 10, 1968, the Defendant refused to speak with the Plaintiff or discuss anything with her and has continued to feel (sic) and refuse to communicate with her. At said time he informed the Plaintiff he wished to live separate and apart from her and that he did not desire to live with her any longer and he desired to live alone or to "go find himself a nice whore."

Appendix B: Amended Bill of Particulars

23. On or about July 17, 1968, the Defendant advised the Plaintiff that he would no longer be responsible for her support and maintenance and/or any of their common expenses or the support of their children and at said time berated, screamed, and cursed the Plaintiff, that he would "come and go as he pleased" and that if she, the Plaintiff, did not like it she could "get out," that he had no further use for her and he did not need her any longer.

24. On July 25, 1968, the Defendant demanded that the Plaintiff leave their common domicile and find a separate place to reside and provided her with the sum of $100.00 to leave.

25. Following the departure of the Plaintiff from the common domicile of the parties, the Defendant made the following false and malicious accusations and statements concerning the Plaintiff: (1) that the Plaintiff did not keep a clean and proper house, (2) that the Plaintiff neglected the children of the parties, (3) that the Plaintiff withdrew all of the funds of the parties from their joint account without the knowledge and consent of the Defendant, (4) that, in August, 1966, the Defendant went to the Plaintiff "on hands and knees" and promised not to resume marital relations with the Plaintiff and that they had been living that way ever since, (5) that the Plaintiff refused to permit the Defendant visitation rights with their daughter, all of which statements were untrue.

███████████████████████
Attorney for Plaintiff

Appendix C: Summary of Golden Living Court Decision

The entire decision and the dissenting opinion by Judge Renee Cohn Jubelirer are available on my website: https://www.wbeerman.com.

The Pennsylvania attorney general's lawsuit accused Golden Living of (1) violations of the Unfair Trade Practices and Consumer Protection Law (UTPCPL), (2) breach of contract, and (3) unjust enrichment.

Regarding the UTPCPL, the court ruled in its 48-page decision that Golden Living did not make false advertising claims for the services it provided, but rather only engaged in "puffery," which it said is not a violation of the UTPCPL. The court said puffery, an exaggeration or overstatement expressed in broad, vague, and commendatory language, is meant to be considered as the seller's opinion only, and is to be discounted as such by the buyer. The court also said the attorney general's complaint was not sufficiently specific and detailed. In addition, the court ruled that the state was legally prohibited from seeking restoration under the UTPCPL.

Regarding the breach of contract issue, the court ruled that the state's relationship with Golden Living "was not contractual in nature," and was based on enrollment forms rather than contracts.

Regarding whether Golden Living was subject to laws about unjust enrichment, the court ruled that the state

Appendix C: Summary of Golden Living Decision

legislature provided other specific alternative remedies regarding billing disputes.

In a five-page opinion, Judge Renee Cohn Jubelirer dissented with parts of the court's decision, saying that a "catch all" provision in the UTPCPL eliminates the need to prove false claims were made in advertisements. Rather, she said, a section of the law gives plaintiffs a cause of action to remedy "any . . . fraudulent or deceptive conduct which creates a likelihood of confusion or of misunderstanding." Jubelirer said, "I would therefore not dismiss this claim . . . insofar as it alleges deceptive conduct involving bills and care plans which could directly impact [ongoing] purchasing decisions."

She also said the Court based part of its decision on an argument not raised by Golden Living: that the attorney general had not attached copies of evidence to the complaint. Because the issue was not raised prior to the decision, the attorney general had no opportunity to respond, or explain why not, she said.

Appendix D: Private Attorneys and Nursing Homes

Although this book focused on broad-scope litigation regarding chains of nursing homes by state attorneys general (AGs), I wanted to mention that private attorneys and law firms put together effective lawsuits on behalf of single clients using some of the same tactics as the AGs.

One such private attorney who I encountered in my research is Melanie Bossie of Scottsdale, AZ, with whom I have no business or personal ties. She took issue with my comment that it can be hard to find an attorney to take a nursing home injury case because elderly people do not have long-term earnings potential and long life expectancies, and therefore, their cases are not seen has having much value, or potential for large settlements or awards.

Ms. Bossie pointed out that her firm has had success on behalf of nursing home residents who were in their nineties.

"Juries look at the conduct of the nursing home," rather than the age of the nursing home resident, she said. Private attorneys can bring in testimony from nursing home employees, results of inspections by oversight agencies, and testimony from nursing home industry experts.

In one case handled by Bossie's firm, Wilkes & McHugh, which operates in multiple states, a jury awarded a $1.6 million compensatory damage verdict on behalf of a 90-year-old nursing home resident from Arkansas. Four former nursing home employees testified that the home was understaffed to the point that employees could not carry out their duties in a timely fashion.

In another Arkansas case, involving a 93-year-old nursing home resident, presentation of the results of two surveys/inspections conducted by the government Office of Long Term Care "inflamed the jury," according to defense lawyers. The inspection results, along with other evidence, led the jury to award $63 million in punitive damages to the resident's family. It was the largest such award in Arkansas history by far. The amount "shocked the court's conscience" and the courts reduced the award by two-thirds – to $21 million.

Ms. Bossie had 53 nursing home cases in litigation and 45 in pre-suit stage in New Mexico when I spoke with her in May 2017. She said she has 18 years of experience in nursing home litigation and 8 years as a prosecutor. The defendants' attorneys "know I am willing to take the case to trial," she said, and 90-95 percent of her cases end up with a successful resolution, she said.

Wilkes & McHugh has represented thousands of families in nursing home cases since 1985. "Initially," said a W&M spokesperson, "although many cases of nursing home abuse and neglect were documented, very few firms would challenge nursing home corporations when they provided bad care."

"Because nursing home abuse and neglect claims often involve the same companies we've faced time and time again, we don't have to spend the time and resources it takes to learn what many other attorneys are discovering for the first time."

Appendix E: Remaining Questions for HHS and CMS

I received mixed responses to questions I submitted to the Centers for Medicare and Medicaid Services (CMS), and to the Department of Health and Human Services (HHS). I received some courteous, timely, and helpful responses during the course of my research from the director of the CMS Center for Clinical Standards and Quality/Survey and Certification Group (SCG); an administrative specialist in the SCG; and the director of the SCG Division of Nursing Homes. I appreciate the time and effort spent on developing those responses; I know the officials are busy. However, some questions that were referred into the Freedom of Information Act system and to CMS regional offices took 8 months to produce a reply, some of the responses were inadequate, or no response was forthcoming in some cases.

In June 2017, just before this book was published, after reflecting on the book's overall contents, I submitted five questions to CMS and to the HHS deputy assistant secretary for public affairs for health care. I received a brief response to the first four questions from SCG, but no reply from the deputy assistant secretary.

In the introduction for the questions for CMS, I said: "Although for questions 1-4 below, the book as currently drafted does not directly correlate problems at the state level with CMS oversight, some readers are likely to wonder about CMS's role and responsibility with regard to these problems. So, would CMS like to respond to the questions below?"

Appendix E: Remaining Questions for HHS and CMS

The reply from SCG was: "Our only comment at this time is that we continue to work with all states on their oversight and performance in nursing home surveys. We're not in a position to comment on generalized or speculative perceptions related to that oversight activity."

The questions follow.

1. Enforcement actions in Pennsylvania dropped from a high of 171 in 2003 to only two in 2012, and then went back up slightly to 14 in 2013, 20 in 2014, and, under a new secretary of health, to 52 in 2015. Should a state's apparent virtual cessation of enforcement actions for a year (2012) and a general substantial reduction over a decade trigger a response from CMS, as an oversight agency? Did CMS notice the drastic drop in enforcement actions, and take any action in response? Pennsylvania also ceased to accept anonymous complaints for 3 years, beginning in July 2012, which, according to the state auditor general, was contrary to CMS [policy]. Does the decrease in enforcement actions in Pennsylvania reflect on CMS's performance in its oversight role?

2. State attorney general lawsuits allege unsatisfactory conditions in [some] nursing homes, staffing shortfalls ranging as high as 70 percent of staffing needed, and multiple instances of nursing homes knowing in advance when inspectors are coming for unannounced inspections. A Pennsylvania newspaper series entitled "Failing the Frail" (Page 197 of the draft book) said the state DOH downplayed the severity of nursing home fatality cases. Do these circumstances reflect on CMS's performance in its oversight role?

3. A GAO report (GAO-16-33) showed consumer complaints were up 21 percent while serious deficiency

Appendix E: Remaining Questions for HHS and CMS

citations by oversight agencies were down 41 percent. Does this reflect on CMS's performance in its oversight role?

4. Data in some CMS reports is a year old or older. The 2015 Nursing Home Data Compendium, which contained data for 2014, was released on March 25, 2016. The 2016 Data Compendium, which presumably will contain data from 2015, is not out as of mid-June 2017. Implementation of the 2010 Affordable Care Act's requirements for reporting of nursing home staffing levels had not fully occurred as of mid-2016. Is CMS sufficiently current in its oversight work?

5. The Secretary of the Department of Health and Human Services, a physician who in the 2015-2016 congressional election cycle received $459,393 in campaign contributions from the health sector, wants to restrict lawsuit awards against the health providers. How much consideration was given to the effect of such restraints on persons injured by health providers and on the quality of health care provided to consumers if the potential consequences to providers for negligence are limited?

In my email to the HHS deputy assistant secretary, I wrote: "I think the matters addressed in the questions deserve more attention, and I believe they are sufficiently important to millions of Americans to merit attention at the HHS Secretariat level. For example, are there restraints on CMS's ability to oversee state oversight agencies effectively, and if so, why not address those restraints?"

I will post any further replies I receive on my website at *https://www.wbeerman.com*

Appendix F: Examples of Supplemental Documents Available at https://www.wbeerman.com

Court Documents

Case	Court	Document	Date	Status
New Mexico Attorney General vs Preferred Care, Inc. and Cathedral Rock Corporation	New Mexico First District Court, Santa Fe	Amended Complaint	April 1, 2015	Ongoing; Trial set for 2018
Pennsylvania Attorney General vs Golden Living	Pennsylvania Commonwealth Court	Amended Complaint	September 8, 2015	Pending Appeal as of May 2017
Pennsylvania Attorney General vs Reliant Senior Care Holdings	Pennsylvania Commonwealth Court	Complaint, Order for Final Judgment by Consent, and Attorney Fee Approval	October 3, 2016	Settled October 2016
Pennsylvania Attorney General vs Grane Healthcare	Pennsylvania Commonwealth Court	Complaint and Petition for Injunctive Relief	November 3, 2016	Withdrawn as of May 2017
Pennsylvania Attorney General vs Golden Living	Pennsylvania Commonwealth Court	Decision and Dissenting Opinion	March 22, 2017	Pending Appeal as of May 2017

Appendix F: Examples of Documents Available

Other Documents

Nursing Home Quality Improvement Task Force Report, Pennsylvania Department of Health, Dr. Karen H. Murphy, Secretary, September 22, 2016

Performance Audit Report, Pennsylvania Department of Health (On Nursing Home Oversight), Department of the Auditor General, Eugene A. DePasquale, Auditor General, July 2016

Audit Report -- ***NURSING HOME QUALITY: CMS Should Continue to Improve Data and Oversight***, GAO 16-33, Government Accountability Office, October 2015

Audit Report – ***NURSING HOMES: Consumers Could Benefit from Improvements to the Nursing Home Compare Website and Five-Star Quality Rating System***, GAO 17-61, Government Accountability Office, November 2016

www.ingramcontent.com/pod-product-compliance
Lightning Source LLC
Chambersburg PA
CBHW052237220526
45471CB00001B/79